Hyperemesis Gravidarum

The Definitive Guide

Caitlin Dean, RGN
Amanda Shortman

ISBN: 978-0-9930623-0-8
1st edition, paperback
Published by Spewing Mummy in 2014
Cover design by Revival Design

Dedication

This book is dedicated to our own hyperemesis gravidarum survivors – Oscar Shortman and Alfie, Patrick and Órlaith Dean. We hope that the work we do now will change the experience of hyperemesis gravidarum for your entire generation. We hope to make you proud.

And to our husbands, Rob Dean and Tim Shortman, without their support this book couldn't have happened.

Acknowledgments

Special thanks go to Dr Tony Barnie-Adshead, his wife Rosemary, and his daughter Caroline; Dr Roger Gadsby; Margaret, Nev and Debbie Fisher; Christine and Stephen Shortman; Dr Margaret O'Hara; Dr Marjory Maclean; Dr Brian Swallow; Dr Catherine Sykes; Susie Nicholas; Helen Hendy; Emma Edwards; the team at the HER Foundation, particularly Ann Marie and Jeremy King and Kimber MacGibbon; Lyle Brooks and Ashli Foshi McCall at Beyond Morning Sickness; the staff at Motherisk; Mat Connelly and Kat Smith at Iteracy; Paul Colledge at Revival Design; Dr Harriet Tulberg; Dr Sophie Haynes; Mandy Bellenger RMN; Emma Moxham RGN; Dr Richard Cockshott and Polly Amos; Kate Hilpern; Heather Miranda; Anaya Carter; Abi and Neil Briggs; Jo Cole; Rupert and Angela Warwick; Joanna Ballard; Kelly Hadaway; and everyone else who has supported us through our pregnancies and through PSS and Spewing Mummy to make this book happen.

How The Book Came To Be

The idea for this book came about due to a lack of accessible information regarding hyperemesis gravidarum. Amanda began writing about the subject during her own pregnancy in 2011 but soon realised that covering it in the detail it deserved was impossible when working to the tight word limits she was given by the general media outlets. And so, when her son was just three months old she began writing the book.

She wanted it to be accessible to anyone suffering from HG whilst still being respected by healthcare professionals, and so she threw herself into the world of medical journals and research papers and devoted many hours to learning all she could about the condition. Needless to say progress on the book was slow, with the first few chapters (so heavily based on research) taking the longest. Realising that the book would take many years to complete on her own, Amanda started to look for a co-author and in 2013 Caitlin came on board.

Having already written extensively on the subject herself, both for the Pregnancy Sickness Support Website and her own blog, Caitlin was the ideal co-author for the book. As a Registered General Nurse, she was able to include information for healthcare professionals to compliment the research based chapters already written. And as a survivor of three HG pregnancies she was able to focus on the chapters dedicated to partners and preparing for another pregnancy whilst Amanda focussed on the post-HG chapters and one child families.

Amanda and Caitlin's respective experiences and professional backgrounds have led to the production of a book that covers everything you need to know about hyperemesis gravidarum and truly is The Definitive Guide.

About the Authors

Caitlin Dean is a Registered General Nurse who has been involved in the hyperemesis gravidarum world for a number of years, having suffered through three of her own pregnancies. She writes prolifically on the subject for both the general press and for medical journals. She has had numerous national TV appearances and radio interviews talking about her experience, representing the charity Pregnancy Sickness Support as a Trustee and discussing research into the field. Considered a voice for the HG community in Britain and abroad she advocates at every opportunity for better care and treatment using the most up to date evidence based research.

You can follow Caitlin's own blog at www.spewingmummy.co.uk

Amanda Shortman is a language graduate with extensive experience of writing for both online media and printed publications. She is also the Volunteer Coordinator for the charity Pregnancy Sickness Support, providing information and support to hundreds of sufferers each year and managing the national network of volunteers. Despite no medical background, Amanda has read vast amounts of research on HG and uses her communication skills to raise awareness of the condition through her writing, attending conferences, and liaising with the media. As a mother to an only child, she is a voice for those who limit their family size due to HG and has spoken of this on national TV.

You can follow Amanda's own blog at www.thefamilypatch.com

Contents

Supporting materials and all charts are available at www.spewingmummy.co.uk

Preface

What Is Hyperemesis Gravidarum, and Why Write a Book About It?

Hyperemesis gravidarum is, on the most basic level, an extreme form of nausea and vomiting in pregnancy (NVP). It is much rarer than the more typical symptoms of nausea and vomiting that many women experience during their first trimester, and very often it is totally omitted from pregnancy-related literature. So you can be forgiven if the term hyperemesis gravidarum (or HG as it is often called by its sufferers) is one you have never heard before.

And yet, though a much smaller proportion of pregnant women suffer from HG, there is a real need for awareness of and support for those suffering from the condition. HG can and usually does turn what many women regard as a fulfilling and joyful time of their lives into the worst nightmare imaginable for its sufferers. The physical symptoms alone are traumatic enough, but the mental and emotional responses to it can be just as devastating.

Amanda's story:

I suffered from severe NVP during my first, and only, pregnancy. I believe I suffered from undiagnosed HG as I lost over 10% of my pre-pregnancy weight, survived on less than 500 ml of liquid a day for several weeks and spent months house-bound (sometimes completely bed-bound) by my symptoms. My care was pretty appalling and completely inconsistent. At 5 weeks, a GP told me he thought it was all in my head but prescribed an anti-emetic (which didn't help), and then a couple of weeks later, a nurse practitioner told me she could see I was clearly dehydrated and instructed me to double the dose of the anti-emetic, only to tell me the following day that because there were no ketones present in my urine, I could not be admitted to hospital for fluids, I shouldn't be taking any medication, and I just had to 'put up and shut up'. From that point onwards, I fought a battle I had little strength for, and it took me until my fifth month to finally be prescribed another anti-emetic, which thankfully helped control my symptoms. I saw almost every GP in my surgery and was told all manner of things, but never given any clear information about what was happening to me. I was told there was nothing I could take to help with my symptoms, and my worry over things like my continued weight loss was dismissed without any attempt to alleviate my concerns. Thankfully, I was lucky enough to come across a US blogger who was also suffering and who empowered me to seek the help I needed and deserved. My sickness continued to the end of the pregnancy but at a much more manageable level once I finally received treatment that worked – I even had a blissful eight weeks during the latter part of my second trimester when if I ate regularly and rested enough, I felt pretty normal. I'll never forget how incredible that felt! I just wish all women were given the information and support they needed right away, without having to fight so hard just to be heard. That's why I started the book. It's why I got involved with the charity Pregnancy Sickness Support, and it's why I continue to fight for change.

Caitlin's story:

I suffered from HG during my three pregnancies. In my first two, the care I received from my doctors was terrible and disjointed. I was brushed off and made to feel silly, selfish, and pathetic. But that was nothing compared to the isolation I experienced. Despite unfaltering support from my husband, no one else understood what I was going through, and I was utterly alone in my suffering. House-bound, in the days before Facebook on smart phones, I was going stir-crazy. Attempts to 'help myself' and get out of the house resulted in violent emetic episodes and days of deterioration. I went through it again with knowledge of medication and hope that support would be better but found that the treatments are no cure and the isolation was even more profound. By my third pregnancy, I had found a better doctor. Early and pro-active treatment kept symptoms under control for the most part, although it was still a challenge to get through every day. The biggest help though was the support I received from fellow sufferers whom I had met online, yet some of my closest friends now. The support network was born via my involvement in Pregnancy Sickness Support, and it has grown from there. My Spewing Mummy Blog has reached out to sufferers to provide a different sort of support – proactive and humorous I hope to inspire people to change the public attitude to hyperemesis, crush the myths that make our suffering worse, and improve care and treatment for sufferers around the world.

And so the reason for this book is twofold: to create an easily accessible source of information on the latest research into HG thereby helping to raise awareness of the condition, and to provide support to those suffering (or recovering) from hyperemesis and their families. The factual information printed in this book is balanced out by personal experiences of those who have faced severe NVP and HG before, in the hope that this will produce a book that helps as many women as possible to get through their pregnancies with the resources they need to make an informed choice about the management of their symptoms.

We'll be covering the topic of HG and severe NVP in much more detail throughout the numerous chapters, providing references to medical research which you can use to help gain the recognition and support you need from your doctor, midwife, or consultant. However, it is not a text book, and so to keep it accessible to the women suffering in a number of areas, we refer to 'studies' collectively, which healthcare professionals (HCPs) may wish to access for themselves to gain a greater understanding. Rather than bombard women with references we have made the assumption throughout the book that healthcare professionals are capable of investigating studies further through their own online library memberships.

We know that one of the most difficult aspects of dealing with such severe pregnancy sickness comes from trying to explain in any kind of adequate detail just what this really means to those you see every day. Whether it's unsympathetic family members, friends who just cannot understand why you have no time for them anymore, or work colleagues and management who put pressure on you to return to work before you're ready. Most women with severe pregnancy sickness complain of someone who seems to have no understanding of what it means to be that ill.

And so, for that reason, we have produced a 'cheat sheet' of the most common and important points about pregnancy sickness that you can tear out and produce as 'evidence' to anyone who questions you or refuses to listen to what you're saying. You can find this at the end of this preface. If you do not wish to tear the page out of the book, you can also download a printable copy from the Spewing Mummy website. We do hope it will help.

Finally, we want to point you to the organisations providing support, particularly the UK-based charity Pregnancy Sickness Support whose details are listed below and in the resource list at the end of the book. The charity is working hard to raise awareness of severe NVP and HG and build up a support network of volunteers around the country. Their aim is to inform rather than advise. They also put an emphasis on the fact that NVP is on a spectrum rather than having very clear and distinct stages and that any woman suffering from NVP that negatively affects her life in any way should be given support. Both of the authors work closely with the charity, and so we hope that we can follow the charity's lead in this book by providing accurate information that benefits not only those with the more extreme form of HG but also those who are suffering from moderate to severe NVP.

Pregnancy Sickness Support (PSS)
Registered Charity No. 1094788
Information Line: 020 7638 2020
www.pregnancysicknesssupport.org.uk

For those outside the United Kingdom, there is information in the appendix about the Hyperemesis Education and Research (HER) Foundation in America and other organisations around the world who can help you. The information in this book is aimed at a UK audience in terms of medication names and the healthcare system structure of the United Kingdom. Much of it will be relevant to other countries too but not all, so it is best to contact the HER Foundation for treatment information specific to your location.

Beyond Morning Sickness is a book written by HG veteran Ashli Foshee McCall as a comprehensive guide to hyperemesis and its treatments. Based in America, the treatments and healthcare system is very different to the United Kingdom, so where this book is relevant to a UK audience Beyond Morning Sickness picks up the pieces for American readers. Caitlin would not have gone through hyperemesis again were it not for Ashli's book, and it was very much the inspiration for this book. We hope this definitive guide for the UK will compliment the books already on the market and we highly recommend *Beyond Morning Sickness*.

You'll also find a number of supporting materials on the Spewing Mummy website which accompanies this book. From survival calendars to download to blog posts about specific symptoms, there are lots of resources on there to help you get through the nightmare of HG. The cheat sheet below is available there along with all the other charts, care plans, and checklists from the book.

www.spewingmummy.co.uk

A note on our desicion to publish independently

Despite discussions with agents and publishers both in the UK and in America we decided to go down the independent route for two main reasons. Firstly and most importantly was control over content. We both felt that unless the editor happened to have been a sufferer themselves they were highly unlikely to understand the importance of much of the book's content, particularly the emotional aspects of hyperemesis support and care. We didn't want what we consider to be the most important aspects of the book to be stripped out or toned down by an editor who has never suffered. Secondly, there is a pretty niche market for hyperemesis gravidarum literature as it's not a hugely common condition so, quite frankly, we'll make more money, much of which will be ploughed back into the HG charities, by self publishing!

Hyperemesis gravidarum is not a "popular" condition to donate money to and the two main international charities, Pregnancy Sickness Support and The HER Foundation both struggle to get the funds to continue their crucial work. Both the authors currently provide significant financial and practical support not just to the UK charity but also to the Hyperemesis Improvement Movement happening all around the world - We need to make that more sustainable. If we published through a traditional publishing house it would be years before we saw a penny for our work. This way we can guarantee that a significant proportion of every book sale will come straight back to the authors and therefore further the work of the International Hyperemesis Improvement Movement by funding their work. Not only will a minimum of 10% of the profit from the book go direct to hyperemesis charities but the remainder will allow the authors to continue dedicating so much time and energy to raising awareness and supporting women.

Finally, by publishing independently the authors retain control over the promotion of the book. Instead of working with a PR team who do not necessarily know the HG Community, the authors are able to work with people dedicated to the cause.

Cheat Sheet

- NVP affects approximately 70–80% of all pregnant women.
- 35% of pregnant women experience symptoms that are of clinical significance.
- 30% of pregnant women require time off work to manage their symptoms.
- It is estimated that up to 1.5% of women suffer from hyperemesis gravidarum (HG)[1].
- The cause of HG remains unknown, and there is no 'cure'. Treatment usually revolves around trying to limit the severity of the symptoms.
- Milder forms of NVP may end between 12 and 16 weeks; however, those with more severe symptoms and HG often report that though the intensity of symptoms may decrease around this time, up to 60% continue to suffer from nausea and/or vomiting until birth.
- 'Morning Sickness' is an erroneous term as most women experience symptoms of nausea and vomiting at various times throughout the day. Pregnancy sickness is a more appropriate term to use.
- The advice to eat 'little and often' may help in milder cases of NVP, but dietary changes are often not enough for more severe forms, especially HG.
- Similarly, the advice to eat such things as ginger and dry crackers may help milder forms of NVP but is often completely irrelevant to a woman who is struggling to keep any food or liquid down.
- Rest is a vital aspect of managing the symptoms of nausea and vomiting as stress and exhaustion can exacerbate symptoms. Therefore, pressure to 'carry on as normal' can make matters worse.
- Symptoms can become so severe that the pregnant woman may experience dehydration, production of ketones, nutritional deficiencies, electrolyte imbalances, and weight loss.
- Admittance to hospital for IV fluids may be necessary.

---

[1] Some studies suggest this is a low estimate given the difficulty in diagnosing HG.

- Prior to the development of IV treatment, HG was a significant cause of maternal death. Although the last deaths in the UK due to complications of HG were in the 1990s, the severity of this condition should not be forgotten or underestimated.

- Anti-emetic medication may be prescribed to try and limit the severity of the symptoms. Though none are currently licensed in the United Kingdom for use during pregnancy, many have been used successfully for decades without any known effect on the foetus.

- Pregnant women whose weight gain is low in association with HG through out their pregnancy have a higher risk of preterm labour, babies with low birth weight, and babies who are small for their gestational age. The risks increase if HG is still uncontrolled or untreated in the second trimester.

- The emotional stress of prolonged and severe nausea and vomiting is high and support is crucial.

- Antenatal depression, postnatal depression, and post traumatic stress dis order may accompany or follow a pregnancy complicated by severe NVP and HG.

- HG can be so traumatic that sufferers may request a termination of their pregnancy and/or decide against further pregnancies.

Hanging over the edge of my bed, stomach acid trickling from my mouth to the bucket on the floor. It burns my torn oesophagus, my tongue, my cracked and dry lips. I've been here for weeks... no months, I think. I haven't seen a soul other than my husband for days. The last person was a doctor. He made me feel weak and guilty. He signed my sick note and handed me a prescription with dire warnings of unknown risks.

My nose is my worst enemy. I smell everything for miles around, warped and distorted. My poor husband banished to the spare room in between helping me empty sick bowls and change wet knickers - the emetic episodes are violent now, and I can't control it.

Inside me, the life I so desperately wanted stirs. All I feel is nausea, sadness, loneliness, and anger. I worry we won't bond. I worry we won't survive. I hate the thoughts running through my head of termination and miscarriage and just desperately wanting to feel well. I feel guilty. I feel ashamed. I feel scared.

I am weak. I am thin. My muscles are wasting away. I can barely walk now and don't have the strength to cry anymore, although sometimes I waste precious liquid with tears that soak into the pillow my head has rested on for uncountable hours now.

This isn't normal, this isn't joyous or beautiful, this can't be helped with ginger... this is hyperemesis gravidarum.

(Caitlin, HG Survivor, Author)

Part I

About Hyperemesis Gravidarum

(Especially for Healthcare Professionals)

CHAPTER 1

What Is Hyperemesis Gravidarum?

Authors' Note: The following chapters are all written with a heavy emphasis on medical research in the hope they will provide both the sufferer and her healthcare team with the information and knowledge they both need to diagnose, treat, and manage her sickness in the best possible way. In order to ensure that these chapters are as accurate and current as possible, academic terms have been used throughout. A glossary of terms has been provided at the end of the book, and a 'cheat sheet' of more basic information can be found in the book's Preface.

Introduction

Hyperemesis Gravidarum (HG) is a condition which causes severe nausea and vomiting during pregnancy, often resulting in hospital admission. Nausea and vomiting during pregnancy (NVP) is considered to affect anywhere between 50–90% of all pregnant women at some point during early pregnancy dependent upon which source is referenced. In comparison to this, the incidence rate of HG ranges from 0.3% to 1.5% of all live births[2]. However, despite this extreme difference between these two rates of incidence, it is still very difficult to pinpoint exactly when severe NVP should be classed as HG as no definitive clinical definitions of HG exist. In addition to this, NVP is considered to cover a wide spectrum of degrees to which it affects a woman's life.

The more common experience of intermittent nausea and the odd bout of vomiting leads to the general belief that NVP is manageable through basic lifestyle changes such as getting adequate rest and eating 'little and often'. And this is indeed enough for many women. But studies show that more than 30% of women require time off work to cope with their symptoms and 35% of all pregnant women experience symptoms which are of clinical significance, with both physical and psychosocial effects.

---

[2] Some studies suggest that this is a low estimate, due to the difficulty in diagnosing HG leaving many cases unreported. The actual incidence rate of Hyperemesis Gravidarum (HG) could be much higher.

Both the more common milder forms of NVP and the more severe forms, including HG, typically begin between the fourth and eighth week of gestation, with the peak of severity around 9 weeks. Current research suggests that these symptoms generally end between the twelfth and twentieth week with only a minority of women continuing to experience symptoms beyond the twentieth week. However, a recent large-scale online survey by Pregnancy Sickness Support (PSS) of women who had suffered from HG suggests that though there is a decrease in the severity of symptoms around this time, the symptoms continue for most, around 60%, until the very end of pregnancy. About 20% of women never even had a reduction of severity from symptoms for the full gestation.

It is crucial therefore that the healthcare providers of any pregnant woman are aware of the need to distinguish between NVP which can be successfully managed with lifestyle and dietary changes and the more severe forms of NVP, including HG, which warrant a more tailored approach.

It is becoming increasingly accepted that the previously common term 'morning sickness' is erroneous as even those women with mild symptoms often report discomfort throughout the day and night. Pregnancy sickness is a far preferable term. Currently, knowledge and understanding of the term HG and the treatment options available remain uncommon, and women with HG are often left undiagnosed and untreated until their symptoms become severe enough to require a hospital admission.

The difficulty for the healthcare provider lies in the fact that no standard definition of HG exists. There are, however, various clinical definitions proposed in several research papers, two of which are shown below:

- *Fairweather (Ismail review)*

According to the Fairweather criteria, hyperemesis gravidarum should be indicated when vomiting is more frequent than three times per day and there is evidence of weight loss, ketosis, and electrolyte imbalance and volume depletion. The typical onset is considered to be between weeks 4 and 8 continuing through to weeks 14–16, although it is noted that continuation of symptoms into the second and third trimesters is not uncommon.

- *The International Statistical Classification of Disease and Related Health Problems ICD-9 Code 643 (Ismail review)*

This code defines hyperemesis gravidarum as persistent and excessive vomiting which starts before the 22nd week of gestation. It provides further subdivisions, suggesting that these symptoms alone should lead to the diagnosis of 'mild' hyperemesis gravidarum, whilst the addition of metabolic disturbances such as carbohydrate depletion, dehydration, and electrolyte imbalance should lead to the diagnosis of 'severe' hyperemesis gravidarum.

These two definitions of HG, though helpful, are rather vague and differ quite substantially from each other. And they are not the only two that exist. So it is possible to see why diagnosing and treating HG can be so difficult. Without any definitive guidelines and very few clinical tests that show an indication of the need for treatment, healthcare providers often have to rely on limited knowledge and experience when trying to decide if a diagnosis of HG should be given and medication prescribed. Combined with the devastating effects of Thalidomide in the fifties and sixties, many remain wary and choose to err on the side of what they consider to be caution, even if that means prolonging the pregnant woman's suffering and in fact could be more risky than treating with safe medications.

This is far from ideal, and there are many authors who believe that treatment should be provided for any level of NVP which substantially affects a woman's quality of life. It is of significant importance that the majority of women report that persistent nausea is far more troubling than the vomiting they experience, though that is of course traumatic. Therefore, care must be taken to ensure that the symptoms a pregnant woman experiences are given appropriate care and attention so that the best possible options for management can be determined.

Treatment options for HG will be discussed further in this book, first though, let's address the current research into pregnancy sickness and HG

How to Tell the Difference Between Normal Pregnancy Sickness and Hyperemesis Gravidarum
Courtesy of Pregnancy Sickness Support

Symptoms	**'Normal' or Mild Pregnancy Sickness**	**Moderate–Severe Pregnancy Sickness**	**Hyperemesis Gravidarum**
Occurrence rates	Around 80% of all pregnant women suffer from pregnancy sickness of some degree	Around 30% of all pregnant women require time off work, & 35% have symptoms of clinical significance	Between 1–2% of all pregnant women will be diagnosed with Hyperemesis Gravidarum
Typical onset and duration of nausea and/or vomiting	Begin around 4–6 weeks, generally ease between 12 and 20 weeks	Begin around 4–6 weeks, may last beyond 12–20 weeks	May begin before pregnancy confirmed, typically peak at 9–13 weeks, but often last throughout entire pregnancy.
Severity of nausea and/or vomiting	Varies, however typically short periods of nausea and infrequent vomiting episodes. Easily managed through lifestyle and diet changes	Will often impact quality of life, with regular nausea and/or daily vomiting episodes while symptoms continue	Nausea often constant, with multiple vomiting episodes per day. Affects ability to eat, drink, and care for self and others.
Weight loss	Minimal, if any	May lose several lbs while symptoms persist	Weight loss is often severe and rapid. > 5% of pre-pregnancy weight is common with Hyperemesis

Clinical Symptoms	None	May suffer from dehydration and weight loss. If left untreated, moderate–severe pregnancy sickness can lead to hyperemesis	Dehydration, weight loss, ketosis, electrolyte imbalances. If left untreated, can lead to other complications
Affect on Quality of Life	Minimal, if any	May need to adapt working pattern, rest more, and accept extra help at home while symptoms persist	Quality of life affected completely. Often bed-bound or house-bound, unable to eat, drink, speak, read, watch TV, cope with bright lights or look after self in any way.
Treatment Options	Changes to diet and lifestyle should be enough. Eating 'little and often', ginger and acupressure may help	Changes to diet and lifestyle may help, but typical advice like ginger and acupressure often ineffective. Anti-emetics may be suggested.	Medical treatment is crucial in attempting to limit the severity of symptoms. Anti-emetics, IV hydration, and steroids may all be considered.
Other considerations	None	Emotional and psychological support may be requested to cope with mental strain of sickness	Antenatal depression, postnatal depression, and post-traumatic stress disorder can be common in women with such severe symptoms

It is important to note that this is a very basic introduction to the differences between 'normal' pregnancy sickness, moderate–severe pregnancy sickness and HG.

The distinction between moderate–severe pregnancy sickness and HG is often unclear.

CHAPTER 2

Proposed Theories and Research into Hyperemesis Gravidarum

Various theories have been presented and studied over past decades, some garnering more support than others. However, no single or combined factors have yet proven to be the exact cause of hyperemesis gravidarum and further research is needed.

Verberg et al. produced an extensive literature review of research into HG between 1966 and 2005 when the review was published. It is well worth reading; however, for ease, in this chapter, we have summarised their findings below. For the purpose of thoroughness and neutrality, we have included all of the theories covered in the literature review, though some have proven to be unlikely causes of HG.

However, we begin this chapter with the theory that we, the authors, feel is the most solid as the actual cause for the symptoms of pregnancy sickness. This is the theory that prostaglandin E2 is the hormone which causes nausea and vomiting of pregnancy from mild to severe. It does not, however, account for why some women are more sensitive to it's emetic effect and develop HG.

HORMONAL THEORIES

Prostaglandin E2

Research by Dr Barnie-Adshead and Dr Gadsby, founders of PSS, looks at the role of the hormone prostaglandin E2. While Barnie-Adshead and Gadsby acknowledge the significant role of human chorionic gonadotrophin (hCG) in causing NVP, their theory is that hCG is a factor which increases the production of prostaglandin E2 (PGE2) from early placental cells and that it is the PGE2 which is the emetic hormone.

They point out that the individual severity of NVP is not always related to the level of her maternal serum hCG. Furthermore, after 14 weeks of gestation, the hCG level in the mother remains fairly constant, but women with hyperemesis or severe NVP can have symptoms lasting beyond 22 weeks and in plenty of cases right to the end of the pregnancy.

In the 1970s, PGE2 was given to induce a termination of pregnancy, but severe nausea and vomiting were consistently found to be a troublesome side effect with some women being affected by nausea and vomiting from far lower doses than other women. The incidence and severity of nausea and vomiting as a side effect of PGE2 even when given as a pessary pre-operatively were so high that it was problematic for the doctors giving anaesthetics for the procedures.

Without giving you a full-blown chemistry lesson, we shall simply say that there is plenty of PGE2 being produced in early pregnancy at the maternal-placental interface (that is where the placenta actually attaches to the mother) and that it is essential to the maintenance of the pregnancy, despite also being used as stimulant for termination. It is involved in the fine balance of immunosuppression required to prevent the mother's cells from invading and attacking the genetically dissimilar baby's cells.

A study by Barnie-Adshead and Gadsby involved taking blood samples from eighteen pregnant women in the community between 7–9 weeks gestation 1) whilst experiencing nausea and 2) at a time, within the same twenty-four-hour period when they were not nauseated. Blood levels of PGE2 was measured along with two other substances, IL-1B and TNFalpha, and related to either the presence or absence of nausea at the time the sample was taken. They found no difference between the levels of IL-1B and TNFalpha between the symptomatic and asymptomatic times, but they found PGE2 was consistently higher at the time the women were nauseated than when they were not. This was independent of the time of day, that is, eight symptomatic samples were before midday and ten were after midday.

The enzyme prostaglandin dehydrogenase (PGDH) is also produced by early placental cells, and this breaks down the PGE2, effectively stopping its emetic capability. PGDH is under the control of progesterone. The amount of PGDH in individual's placentas can vary widely. If progesterone is raised, so too is PGDH, and PGE2 is therefore lowered and the levels of NVP could be expected to decrease. Equally, when treated with an anti-progesterone, the level of PGDH goes down, the PGE2 therefore goes up, and the level of nausea and vomiting can be expected to increase. This has been found to be the case in clinical settings where anti-progesterone treatments are given.

This theory helps to explain the variation of symptoms from woman to woman, the episodic nature of 'normal' pregnancy sickness, and the cessation of symptoms for the majority of women and is certainly the most solid theory we have found. However, further research is needed to expand on this initial study. Furthermore, the significant variation in women's individual responses to PGE2 is not yet explained and warrants investigation.

HCG

HCG is often stated as the most likely cause of HG for two reasons: first, the onset of symptoms typically coincides with the time during pregnancy when hCG levels are at their highest, and second, because there is a higher incidence rate of HG in pregnancies associated with elevated hCG levels such as twin and molar pregnancies and those with a female foetus.

Verberg et al. found twenty-three studies which investigated the relationship between hCG and HG, fifteen of which had been published since 1990 and eleven of these showed significantly higher levels of hCG in HG patients than in controls. Each of these studies were prospective comparative studies, that is they identified subjects who were matched for various reasons (i.e. eight out of the fifteen studies were matched for gestational age) and the differences became a focus for examination.

Supporters of this theory have suggested that the variances in result between the eleven that showed higher levels of hCG and the four that didn't could be caused by differences in the assay methodology used. Diversity in assays has been used, and these can differ in their ability to detect hCG subunits, isoforms, or metabolites. Furthermore, it has been proposed that specific isoforms of hCG may cause HG.

Despite this it is unclear what role hCG levels actually play in regards to HG, and a causal relationship cannot be concluded. Other conditions associated with high hCG levels do not typically result in nausea and vomiting, and those women whose symptoms continue beyond the first trimester when hCG levels are dropping suggest that hCG is not the sole factor in the aetiology of HG. Furthermore, a high hCG pregnancy does not always result in HG.

Progesterone

Researchers have looked for an association between HG and progesterone levels due to the fact that the hormonal activity of the corpus luteum is at its highest in the first trimester when HG is more common. However, results have been somewhat conflicting, with some studies showing significantly higher levels of progesterone in patients with HG when compared with controls and others showing significantly lower levels. Other studies have failed to find any clear correlation between HG and progesterone levels and, due to the small numbers of patients included in these studies and the addition of patients with typical NVP as well as HG, the results have been unconvincing.

A further challenge to the role of progesterone in HG is provided by the fact that pregnancies with elevated levels of progesterone, such as those with multiple corpora lutea, and those where progesterone is administered for luteal phase support, do not exhibit an increased risk of developing HG. This in fact helps to corroborate the Barnie-Adshead theory mentioned above about the role of progesterone in reducing NVP by controlling production of prostaglandin dehydrogenase.

Oestrogens

There are theories that oestrogens may be causally related to HG. These developed due to the higher incidence rate of HG in conditions with high oestrogen levels (such as a higher body mass index and first pregnancies) and the fact that nausea is a common side effect of oestrogen treatments.

There are several ways in which oestrogen could affect the level of nausea and vomiting experienced by pregnant women. High oestrogen levels cause slower intestinal transit time and gastric emptying and may alter the pH balance in the gastrointestinal tract (GIT) which in turn may lead to the development of Helicobacter pylori infection (which is covered later in the chapter). Both of these effects of high oestrogen levels can result in gastrointestinal symptoms including nausea and vomiting.

Several studies have been published in an attempt to look at estradiol (E_2) levels in patients with HG. Although a couple of these found significantly elevated mean oestrogen levels in patients with HG, only one found elevated E_2 levels and other studies failed to confirm these findings

Other pregnancy-specific oestrogens, such as estriol (E_3), have also been considered, but two prospective cohort studies found no difference in the levels of E_3 in women suffering from NVP and none have been published which studied E_3 levels in women with HG.

However, in a retrospective study, a strong correlation was observed between women who suffered from nausea during pregnancy and nausea during use of oral contraceptives. This supports the hypothesis that patients with HG may be more sensitive to the side effects of oestrogens.

Despite the correlations found in some studies between oestrogen levels and symptoms of nausea and vomiting, there are other factors which must be considered. Oestrogen levels rise progressively throughout pregnancy, whilst HG is more prevalent during the first trimester and generally reduces in severity the further through pregnancy a woman gets. Furthermore, oestrogen levels are very high when controlled ovarian stimulation (COS) is used during assisted reproductive techniques (ART), yet there has been no correlation found between incidence rates of HG and those women who have undergone this procedure. Therefore, elevated oestrogen levels and their potential side effects are not considered a satisfactory explanation of HG.

Thyroid Hormones

The thyroid gland is stimulated during early pregnancy, sometimes leading to a state known as gestational transient thyrotoxicosis (GTT), which has been observed in up to two-thirds of women with HG. Several prospective comparative studies have been conducted to compare either the T_4 or TSH levels in women with HG with those of asymptomatic controls. The large majority of these showed significantly higher levels in women with HG than the controls.

There are various ways in which thyroid function may be altered during pregnancy, including the structural similarity between hCG and TSH, which can cause excessive stimulation of the thyroid gland. This has led to the theory that the high incidence of hyperthyroidism in patients with HG could be caused by elevated levels of hCG, thyroid receptors that are hypersensitive to hCG, or the production of a type of hCG that is more potent at stimulating the thyroid gland.

Hyperthyroidism has also been associated with the severity of HG, with one study showing that patients with HG with hyperthyroidism were more likely to experience abnormal electrolyte levels, increased liver enzyme levels, and more severe vomiting.

However, despite many studies showing a relationship between hCG levels and GTT, there is little evidence to suggest the role this has in HG. Hyperthyroidism is not exclusive to patients with HG, and other causes of it (e.g. Graves' disease) do not cause nausea and vomiting.

Leptin

Elevated leptin levels have been observed in several pregnancy-related conditions including pre-eclampsia and gestational diabetes mellitus; however, prospective cohort studies comparing the leptin levels between patients with HG and controls have shown no significant difference. Supporters of this theory have suggested that this could be a false negative finding due to the negative energy balance in patients with HG as dramatic decreases in leptin levels have been observed in other conditions where negative energy balances occur, such as starvation.

Adrenal Cortex

The theory that adrenal cortex insufficiency may be involved in HG developed after Wells observed a reduction of symptoms in patients with HG following treatment with corticosteroids. The insufficiency could be caused by either insufficient ACTH or the inability of the hypothalamic-pituitary-adrenal axis to respond to increased demands for adrenal output in early pregnancy.

Increased ACTH and cortisol levels have also been observed in woman with anorexia and bulimia nervosa, suggesting that it may be a protective mechanism to conserve energy during starvation.

Research into this has been inconclusive, with studies that have observed both elevated and decreased serum cortisol levels. There appears to be a link between the hypothalamic-pituitary-adrenal-cortex and HG; however, it remains unclear whether it is actually involved in the development of HG.

Growth Hormone and Prolactin

Changes in the levels of human growth hormone (hGH) and prolactin have been reported in several studies observing women with both HG and NVP. Some studies have shown production of these two hormones in extra-pituitary tissues (e.g. the endometrium) during pregnancy. This has led to the suggestion that changes in the levels of these two hormones in patients with HG may reflect endometrial and placental production rather than changes in the pituitary gland secretions. Further study is needed to establish what role these changes play in patients with HG.

Placental Serum Markers

Schwangerschafts protein 1 (SP1) is a protein produced by the placenta during the earliest weeks of pregnancy and is used as a marker in the screening for Down's Syndrome. A prospective cohort study to examine the predictive effect of these markers found that SP1 levels seemed to correlate with vomiting during pregnancy. However, a later study could not confirm this.

Immunology Theories

As changes occur in the immune system during pregnancy, it has been suggested that the pregnancy-related disorders may be caused by physiological changes in the immune response of pregnant women.

Several studies have observed elevated levels of several immunological factors in women with HG when compared to controls, including the concentration of foetal DNA in the plasma of pregnant women, immunoglobulin levels, and lymphocyte count. Research has also shown a positive correlation between immunological changes and hormonal changes during pregnancy.

However, starvation normally causes suppression of immune systems, whereas research seems to suggest that there is an activated immune system in patients with HG. It is impossible to determine whether these changes in the immune response are a cause or effect of HG based on the evidence currently available, and the significance of the correlated changes in hormone levels remains unclear.

GASTROINTESTINAL TRACT THEORIES

Helicobacter Pylori Infection

There have been numerous studies that have looked at H. pylori infection in patients with HG, the majority of which have shown a significant increased infection rate in those with HG compared to controls.

Verberg et al. noted, 'Only one study used histological examination of mucosal biopsy, considered to be the gold standard of testing for H. pylori as a diagnostic tool'. However, this study recorded 95% of women with HG as testing positive for H. pylori, compared to 50% of asymptomatic controls. They also found that the density of H. pylori might explain the difference between normal NVP and HG as it seemed to correlate to the severity of symptoms experienced.

This relationship is supported further by reports of women with HG who have not responded to standard treatment for HG but have experienced a complete relief from symptoms following treatment for H. pylori infection.

However, these findings do not explain why many women with H. pylori infection remain asymptomatic and further research is needed.

Gastric and Intestinal Mobility

During pregnancy, many women experience nausea connected to the slower small intestinal and colonic transit times and slow gastric emptying. This abnormal activity in the gastric and intestinal system is caused by changes in the levels of oestrogens and progesterone during pregnancy, particularly towards the end of pregnancy.

It has been suggested that this may relate to HG. However, a study to compare the gastric emptying times in patients with HG and controls actually measured an increase in gastric emptying in patients with HG.

Lower Oesophageal Sphincter Pressure

As many women suffer from gastrointestinal reflux during pregnancy, it has also been suggested that the decrease in lower oesophageal sphincter pressure (LESP) may be connected to HG. However, there is little evidence to support this hypothesis, and as the decrease in LESP tends to occur towards the end of pregnancy when HG is generally less severe, there isn't much support for this theory.

The third trimester relapse which women with HG commonly report could be a result of this.

Fluid Secretion in the Gastrointestinal Tract

Fluid secretion is seen regularly during pregnancy, such as in the case of the production of amniotic fluid. It is also seen in other circumstances such as hydatidiform mole, ovarian hyperstimulation syndrome, and polycystic ovary syndrome, all conditions related to high gonadotrophin levels. There is evidence to suggest that gonadotrophins may affect ion transport and passive fluid movement, leading to the theory that HG may result from the distention of the upper gastrointestinal tract (GIT) caused by excessive fluid secretion and accumulation in the gut lumen.

Studies have shown high-affinity hCG binding sites in the pancreas and duodenum of rats, where much of the GIT secretions originate; however, at the time of the literature review, no studies had been carried out to test the hypothesis on human patients with HG.

METABOLIC ENZYMES THEORIES

Liver Enzymes

Liver function abnormalities have been reported in up to 67% of patients with HG and have been associated with a later onset of HG, more severe ketonuria, and hyperthyroidism. Diagnostic tests including ultrasonography and liver biopsy have shown no abnormal features, and liver enzymes return to normal upon the cessation of vomiting and when adequate nutrition is achieved.

This all suggests that liver enzyme abnormalities are a result of HG rather than a cause of it.

Amylase

Elevated serum amylase has been observed in patients with HG; however, all of these patients had normal pancreatic amylase levels. This suggests that the elevated serum amylase levels are caused by an excessive salivary gland and therefore a result of HG rather than a cause.

NUTRITIONAL DEFICIENCIES THEORIES

Vitamin Deficiency

Early reports mention pyridoxine (vitamin B6) deficiency in relation to HG, and vitamin B6 is currently used in many treatment protocols for HG. However, studies have been unable to show a relationship between this and the incidence or degree of NVP, and no studies have been identified that test the theory on patients with HG.

Deficiencies in other vitamins, including thiamine and vitamin K, have been observed in patients with HG. These may be explained by a combination of increased demands during pregnancy, the absence of nutritional intake, and malabsorption during HG. Similar symptoms have been reported in patients with severe starvation and bulimia nervosa, suggesting that these deficiencies are a result of excessive vomiting in HG rather than the cause. Thiamine is also a commonly prescribed drug in HG treatment protocols because of two deaths of women in the United Kingdom in the 1990s following the development of Wernicke's encephalopathy, a result of thiamine deficiency caused by excessive vomiting.

Trace Element Deficiency

Various studies to investigate the levels of trace elements such as magnesium, copper, and zinc have been carried out but no direct correlation has yet been found. No abnormalities have been observed in magnesium concentrations in patients with HG. Copper concentrations have been found to be low in one study yet normal in another, and zinc levels have been found to be significantly lower in one study, normal in a second, and significantly higher in a third.

Despite the lack of a clear correlation between these trace elements and HG, Verberg et al. suggest that 'a causal relationship cannot be completely excluded' due to the key roles zinc and copper play in regulating metabolic, hormonal, and endocrine functions of several organs.

Anatomy Theories

It has been proposed that women could be more prone to HG due to anatomical variations. This theory has come from the finding that a right-sided corpus luteum has been observed significantly more frequently in a cohort study of patients with NVP. A possible explanation for this could be the difference in venous drainage between the left and right ovary, causing a higher concentration of sex steroids if the corpus luteum is situated on the right side.

However, this theory was not supported by the observation of a woman with severe HG who continued to suffer from symptoms following the excision of a right-sided corpus luteum at 12 weeks.

Furthermore, women who have conceived via IVF have the same risk of HG and yet would not have produced a corpus luteum.

Psychosocial Theories

Psychological and social stress factors have been suggested as a cause for HG for many decades, despite the clear biological connection to pregnancy as indicated by the typical time of onset (fourth-eighth week of gestation) and time of relief from symptoms (often by twentieth week and always after birth). Theories of a psychosocial cause of HG became popular during the twentieth century along with the development of psychoanalytical theory in general. As with many health conditions with an unknown aetiology, HG has suffered from theories based on social suggestions rather than scientific evidence. The very fact that biological causes have not yet provided a satisfactory explanation for HG has enabled these theories to continue to be so popular. (Although the authors would argue that the Barnie-Adshead and Gadsby theory of prostaglandin E2 as a biological cause goes a long way in providing such a satisfactory explanation.)

However, psychosocial theories are relatively modern. O'Brien and Newton created a historical review of beliefs about NVP and found that three distinct eras appeared which they termed the 'Early Somatic Era' (until 1929), the 'Intrapsychic Era' (1930–1980), and the 'Metabolic and Sociological Stress Era' (1981 – present).

The Early Somatic Era seems to date back thousands of years, with nausea and vomiting being described on papyrus that is approximately 4,000 years old. During this era, most records of NVP consisted of observations of its symptoms and possible causes based on physiological changes in the body.

Aristotle made many observations, including that most pregnant women would suffer from nausea and headaches and that symptoms could be present as early as 10 days after the suppression of menses. He also noted that many women experienced relief when the menses were channelled to the breasts where it became milk. It was also a common belief that nausea and vomiting was likely to be worse if the foetus was female.

Between 98 and 138 CE Soranus' Gynaecology included a definition of NVP, and Soranus also observed that the previous suggestions of an increase in NVP if the foetus was female may be incorrect as 'sometimes one thing, sometime the opposite, has resulted'. Yet despite these observations, possible causes for NVP were rarely proposed.

From the 1600s to approximately 1929, scientific enquiry into the cause of NVP looked closely at physiological changes observed in pregnant women, including some post-mortem examinations. From this, two aetiological theories developed: the first being that NVP is caused by a reflex associated with pregnancy and the second being that it is caused by some toxin.

The reflex theory suggested that the sickness experienced during pregnancy was caused by reflex irritation from the growing womb, and the toxin theory suggested undigested food, sperm, and the foetus itself as possible causes.

Although some authors suggested a neurological cause for NVP prior to 1929, it wasn't until this time that severe forms of NVP were generally regarded as being psychological in cause. O'Brien and Newton's 'Intrapsychic Era' led the way for the original theory that sickness was caused by the woman's unconscious loathing of her husband and expected child and an attempt of her unconscious mind to rid herself of the foetus. Interestingly, this coincided with the development of intravenous (IV) therapy, in the early 1930s at which point a dramatic drop in deaths caused by HG was seen.

Though this theory is not commonly accepted today, many other psychological causes have been proposed including immaturity of the mother, lower intelligence, ambivalence about the pregnancy, and conflict about self-image. It has even been suggested that NVP is unique to human mothers; however, this is open to question as observations have been made of other mammals vomiting during pregnancy. Vets report seeing a drop in food intake in domestic dogs during early weeks of pregnancy which could indicate nausea.

The Intrapsychic Era also gave way to the work of Fairweather, whose work is still cited in research papers today, despite questions over the accuracy of his findings. It was his paper that, according to O'Brien and Newton, 'has embedded in the literature the belief that moderate to severe NVP is associated with hysterical personality types and lower intelligence'.

This belief led to the appalling treatment of women during this era, with nurses being instructed to remove the vomit bowl from the patient's view, allow the patient to vomit over herself, and to be in no great hurry to change her.

However, most patients with HG are quick to contend that any symptoms which may be attributed to a mental or emotional state are in fact a result of HG rather than a cause of it. The physical stress of coping with intractable nausea and multiple vomiting episodes per day coupled with the isolation caused by trying to avoid triggers such as movement, sound, and smells could easily lead to trauma and depression. Fortunately, many researchers have begun to record such findings themselves, and though psychosocial beliefs still exist in some parts, they are no longer the only theories presented.

Since the 1980s we have seen a return to scientific research into a variety of the biological mechanisms which may be contributing causes in the development of both NVP and HG. It has been termed by O'Brien and Newton as the Metabolic and Sociological Stress Era, and the majority of the theories and research described earlier in this section fall into this category. It has also led to the observations of various factors which may make a woman more likely to suffer from HG, some of which are listed below:

Risk Factors

- Previous history of HG
- Mother or sister who suffered from HG
- Multiple gestation
- Previous or current molar pregnancy

In comparison to this, smoking is associated with a reduction in the risk of suffering HG, and maternal smoking prior to pregnancy is a significant protective factor against nausea and vomiting, even after considering maternal age and parity. As nausea and vomiting are generally considered to be connected to a well-functioning placenta, this trend may reflect the negative effect of maternal smoking on early placenta development. Smoking is well established as harmful for both the mother and developing foetus and should be avoided in pregnancy.

It should also be noted that whilst nausea and vomiting can be a good sign in pregnancies with typical NVP where it may signal a healthy and well-functioning placenta, care must be taken to avoid devaluing the negative effects of severe NVP and HG which, when left untreated and unrecognised, can cause distress, low weight gain or weight loss, dehydration and electrolyte imbalance.

Genetic Research

A familial history is already an established risk factor with numerous studies finding an increase of 35% for women whose mother or sisters suffered HG. There is exciting research happening in America now looking to isolate a genetic mutation as a cause for HG. Researchers are collecting saliva samples from women who experienced severe hyperemesis, requiring hospital treatment, and saliva from control cases who have had at least two normal pregnancies. They are attempting to isolate genes or risk factors associated with the condition which could explain why some women get HG rather than normal pregnancy sickness. Although isolating a specific gene would not necessarily get us closer to treatment, it would certainly give a lot of women around the world reassurance about their condition. Conditions which do not have a definitive cause are often overlooked by medical communities and researchers, and isolating the cause of HG would increase the awareness and credibility of the condition. That in itself would pave the way for further research into treatments for the symptoms.

CHAPTER 3

For Healthcare Professionals

A woman's experience of hyperemesis gravidarum and her ability to 'survive' the ordeal, with her mental health intact can be significantly affected by her interactions with the healthcare professionals (HCPs) she comes in contact with. A planned study by the authors and the leading HG charities includes looking at the long term psychological impact of the positive and negative support provided by women's HCPs. We hypothesise, from our collective experiences with thousands of sufferers, that women who are treated with dignity and empathic support suffer less post-natal anxiety and trauma in relation to their HG compared to women who suffer negative experiences with seeking help from HCPs. We also hypothesise that positive HCP experiences are less likely to result in women limiting their family size, enabling them to go on to have better planned future pregnancies with better controlled symptoms. However this will require a longer term study to investigate fully.

Sadly, bad practice and treatment based on old wives' tales still prevail in some settings, particularly when it comes to pregnancy. Poor practice witnessed by students is perpetuated when they hear from experienced staff that 'it's all in her head' or 'these hyperemesis patients don't even try to help themselves'. Worse still, are offensive notions that it's a mental rejection of the baby or a symptom of domestic violence which can still today be heard, whispered behind patients' backs in a 'knowing way'. As noted in the previous chapter, such beliefs in a psychosocial cause of hyperemesis are outdated and highly questionable, although still frequently heard by women today. The poor treatment of women based on these views can lead to negative mental and emotional outcomes, as we will discuss in later chapters. It is crucial that such practice is challenged by pro-active professionals so that patients are always treated with the compassion and dignity they deserve during an incredibly difficult time in their lives.

A further challenge faced by women with hyperemesis is an unfounded belief, even amongst HCPs, that no medication is safe in pregnancy; however this is not what the evidence base shows. It is beyond the scope of this book to discuss the full evidence base for all the different options available, and the body of research is constantly growing and developing. You are better off researching your evidence through your own professional online libraries. Charities like PSS and The HER Foundation provide mountains of references to articles and research which may help if you are unsure where to start. Within this book, we do discuss the current dominant treatments in the United Kingdom, but due to the nature of publishing and research, this could have changed by the time of print. However for a good overview, see Chapter 4 for more information on treatment and management of hyperemesis.

So, given the above, what can HCPs do to improve the experience of women with hyperemesis?

Appreciate the Difference Between 'Morning Sickness' and Hyperemesis Gravidarum

Morning sickness or, as we should now refer to it, pregnancy sickness is a normal part of pregnancy, affecting around 80% of pregnant women. It's not particularly nice, but it's not that bad either. Generally it consists of a bit of a queasy feeling sporadically during the day or night, particularly if you haven't eaten. Occasionally it includes vomiting and then feeling a bit better afterwards. Believe it or not, most women actually look forward to this normal part of pregnancy as a sort of 'rite of passage'. It's an indication and reminder of the pregnancy which she has planned and is excited about and it is generally considered a sign of a healthily progressing pregnancy.

Normal pregnancy sickness is usually over by 12 or 14 weeks and can be eased by self-help techniques such as rest and eating little and often. Taking a capsule of ginger extract, 1,000 mg per day may help however ginger biscuits, ginger tea, ginger cordial, or any other ginger product is very unlikely to help other than via the placebo effect and there is no evidence-base to support the suggestion of these.

Women are unlikely to lose significant weight with normal pregnancy sickness, and it should not interfere with their ability to go to work or look after their household. It may, to the sufferer, feel awful but ultimately it's not that bad in the scheme of things, and we all know 'it's worth it in the end'. Most women with normal pregnancy sickness won't express concerns about it and are unlikely to present to a GP or hospital. Women with normal pregnancy sickness don't suffer significant emotional upset or long-term complications from it (with the exception of pre-existing disorders, such as women with emetophobia).

This is the typical experience of pregnancy sickness that most women expect and which most HCPs refer to when they tell pregnant women that being sick during pregnancy is 'normal'. And yet, as stated above, very few women will approach their HCP unless their experience is beyond that which they expected. So the fact that they have even made an appointment to speak to someone should indicate that their symptoms need assessing. It is very difficult to pinpoint exactly when a pregnant woman may need treatment; however, we hope the information below will provide a clear guide on assessing the severity of symptoms. Please also refer to the table at the end of Chapter 1 for a better understanding of the differences between normal pregnancy sickness, moderate–severe pregnancy sickness, and HG.

Pregnancy sickness is on a spectrum from the very mild to the life-threatening. Somewhere around the moderate–severe end of NVP, before it can be fully considered HG, treatment is needed. Whilst it may be difficult to know exactly where on the spectrum a woman may be, if the nausea is so constant that she is unable to eat and drink normally, then she needs treatment. If she is having time off work and is house or bed-bound, then she needs treatment. Without adequate treatment, moderate–severe NVP can become HG.

In many cases, the first-line treatment of antihistamine (i.e. cyclizine or promethazine) plus vitamin B6 will be effective and enable her to gain control over eating and drinking to prevent further deterioration. The vast majority of women, particularly if the pregnancy was planned, do NOT want to take medication in pregnancy. Fears over safety and the impact on the baby may be overwhelming her as she takes that first tablet. GPs, nurses and midwives can reassure her and comfort her by discussing the evidence for their safety and helping her to understand what is meant by terms like risk.

Sadly, the authors hear too many cases where the GP, nurse or midwife has added significant stress and worry with comments such as 'Well, you really shouldn't take anything in pregnancy. We don't know if it's safe'. Qualified staff should be more than capable of accessing and reviewing the relevant literature via online libraries. The idea that 'these women just want to pop a pill to not feel sick' is nonsense yet heard a number of times whilst researching this book and in a PSS study in 2013. To reduce these attitudes amongst professionals we need to challenge our colleagues and lead the way with teaching sessions and printed information.

When severe NVP gets worse and a woman becomes dehydrated, then she has HG and probably needs admission for fluids and IV anti-emetics. Criteria to look for include weight loss greater than 5% of pre-pregnancy weight, dehydration and starvation measured either by fluid intake less than 500 ml/24 hours or ketosis, and quality of life that is severely affected such as being unable to get out of bed, wash, watch TV, read, and so on.

If a woman has HG, then she needs treatment; if not treated, it may lead to serious complications for both mum and baby. Women should be reassured that in a risk verses benefit assessment, taking the medication is the safer option. Another misnomer is that there are no risks to mum or baby if hyperemesis is not treated. This could not be further from the truth. Before the days of modern treatment, it was the leading cause of death in early pregnancy. It is thanks to modern medicine that this is no longer the case although long before death there are numerous other complications that can arise from HG being left untreated. Placental abruption, small for date babies, malnutrition, premature labour, oesophageal tears and ruptures, and significant mental health issues to name but a few, can occur when a woman is left untreated into the second trimester. Furthermore, there is a lack of research into the long-term impact on the foetus of a malnourished and dehydrated mother and the consequences of ketones concentrated in the amniotic fluid.

There are a number of treatment options to move on to after the first line of antihistamine/B6, and adding in rather than switching medication is generally more effective as the various anti-emetics work in different ways. Starting early is also considered to be more effective than waiting until the sickness is very severe, much like taking travel sickness medication before you get in the car/ferry/plane or dosing early with anti-emetics for post operative nausea. Treatment options are discussed in chapter 4 and up to the minute information is available via the websites given in the appendix.

SUPPORTING A WOMAN WITH HYPEREMESIS GRAVIDARUM

Believing Her

Many pregnant women have never heard of HG before and struggle to make friends and family take their symptoms seriously. It is therefore vital that healthcare providers do not question the authenticity of women's symptoms. A 2010 study actually found that unhelpful attitudes from healthcare providers prevented women accessing timely intervention as their symptoms were under-appreciated. Such attitudes can invalidate the concerns of a woman with severe pregnancy sickness, leaving her feeling like she has no choice but to suffer alone and continue trying the typical suggestions to "eat little and often" and "try ginger" which have so far remained ineffective.

In 2013 Margaret O'Hara conducted a qualitative study of women's experiences of HG in relation to healthcare professionals and found that women were frequently offered "folkloric" remedies. The study found that 96% of sufferers were already aware of complementary and alternative therapies. Many women are bombarded by suggestions for 'morning sickness' remedies by relatives and friends, who without medical knowledge are compelled to suggest everything from acupuncture to homeopathy and every herb and crystal in between. As such, when a pregnant woman approaches her GP or midwife regarding the severity of her sickness, it is with trust that the healthcare professional will be able to offer more substantial information and support. However, numerous studies have found that pregnant women are being told inaccurate information, such as HG always ends at 12 weeks and ginger products are the cure for severe symptoms. And inaccurate information by healthcare professionals has been found to directly cause a mistrust of healthcare professionals and a breakdown of the doctor-patient relationship. Therefore it is vital that information given to a pregnant woman suffering from moderate-severe pregnancy sickness and HG is evidence-based and followed up with a discussion regarding the medical treatment options available. Providing information to relatives and friends if they accompany a pregnant woman to a consultation or visit her in hospital is also a great way of spreading awareness and accurate information about the condition and its treatments. The charities mentioned in the appendix provide printable information, and Chapter 8 of this book is specifically for friends and relatives. You are welcome to photocopy it or download it as a leaflet from the Spewing Mummy website.

Advocacy

During my nurse training, I was taught that the nurse should be an advocate for the patient who is unable to express themselves. Yet I've come across many nurses and midwives who feel too intimidated by doctors and consultants to speak up for patients, and I've never really understood why. The doctors themselves admit they do not, indeed cannot, know everything about everything and the vast majority are genuinely pleased if a nurse has a thorough knowledge of a subject. Our roles are different, and most doctors really respect the professional knowledge of the nurses and midwives they proudly call colleagues. So speak up!

(Caitlin, Author)

Women suffering from HG struggle to advocate for themselves and may need help with this, particularly in accessing local services and this is a key role of nurses and midwives. In increasing areas of the UK services such as IV fluids at home and day units for IV rehydration are becoming available. However the pregnant woman may be totally unaware of such options and so informing her when they are available and how she can access these services can make a big difference. Providing information about Pregnancy Sickness Support (PSS), a national charity which provides peer support to sufferers of HG, may also help to empower the sufferer, especially in terms of advocating for herself.

One of the hardest situations to deal with is if a woman has been asked if the baby was 'planned', with the implication that unplanned equals unwanted. This is inappropriate on many levels, not least of which because it suggests a psychosocial cause to the symptoms, which we have clearly seen is an outdated theory. Whether the pregnancy was planned or not, the physical symptoms the woman is experiencing are the same and so the question is unhelpful and unnecessary. The question can also imply that termination may be an option, even when other treatment options have not been considered.

If the prescriber she sees isn't sure of the best way forward, you could suggest they try contacting the charities listed in the appendix. Many doctors are not aware of the current treatments for hyperemesis, particularly for the more severe cases where the more common first and second line treatments have been ineffective. So providing the doctor with sources of information and thereby aiding in the doctor-patient discussions about options may make a huge difference to the suffer.

I just wanted someone to speak up for me. I wanted someone to explain to the doctor that I wasn't making myself sick and I didn't want to take medication but I felt like I'd been poisoned and I couldn't move without retching. I wanted to explain that I had tried so hard for this baby and wanted to keep it more than anything but I felt like I was dying and I was scared. I wanted someone to say to the doctor 'she's scared'. The nurses saw how ill I was, I just wanted them to explain it to the doctor because I was too weak and sick to talk.

(Amy, HG Survivor)

If a woman you're supporting is facing termination solely because of hyperemesis, your role in ensuring she has exhausted all treatment options available is crucial. She may not know all of her options, or she may need help asking for them. It's terribly sad when we hear, surprisingly often, of women terminating babies they desperately wanted without ever being told about the various treatment options. Even harder to hear are the experiences of those who have been refused common treatments, such as ondansetron or steroids, in favour of termination. It's miserable when they get in touch with us afterwards and realise there were other things they could have tried if only they had been offered.

In the UK the termination rate for hyperemesis is nearly 10% but it is a decision that many women regret having had to make. Discovering afterwards that there may have been something else they could have tried, which could have made the difference between continuing and terminating a much-wanted pregnancy, can be very distressing. Often they have come in contact with dozens of HCPs and certainly two doctors will have had to agree to the termination, so it is understandable that they question why no one helped them or told them about the treatments that could have been offered.

However, sometimes a termination is still the choice a woman and her family decide to make, and we discuss this more in chapter 9; however, any woman faced with hyperemesis and discussing termination, for whatever reason, is in a vulnerable position and will likely appreciate an advocate to help her explore her options, even if that is just for controlling symptoms until the procedure.

Distressing Symptoms

Unfortunately, nausea and vomiting are not the only distressing symptoms women with HG experience. In addition to the heightened sense of smell, other delights that come hand in hand with HG include excessive saliva production (called ptyalism), trouble maintaining continence during emetic episodes and constipation, particularly if being treated with ondansetron and exacerbated by dehydration.

Ptyalism, in particular, is reported as a very distressing symptom as women find they have to continuously spit into a cup or towel. Swallowing the saliva is not an option as it can trigger more vomiting, and women report that they find this very embarrassing. If admitted to a ward, ensuring that a woman has an opaque vessel to spit into or a stack of towels available will help. She may also need a towel on her pillow when she sleeps or if she feels too weak to sit up.

Urinating during vomiting can also seem highly humiliating for pregnant women as, until that point, young women tend to think of incontinence pads as the domain of the elderly. A survey conducted via the PSS website in 2013 found that 51% of 769 women asked experienced episodes of incontinence induced by emetic episodes. Of the 51% who experienced it, we asked how distressing they found it on a scale of 0-10, (0 not distressing, 10 very distressing). 64% rated it 6-10 for distress caused and 31% rated it 10 out of 10 (Unpublished report by Pregnancy Sickness Support). Reassuring her that there are products available to use and that it is very common in hyperemesis pregnancies will help with the distress it can cause. Also let her know that it's not permanent, and she will be continent again after the baby is born. Providing information on pelvic floor exercises might be helpful.

Constipation can be particularly bad for patients with HG due to a combination of dehydration, malnutrition, immobility, and standard pregnancy hormones. But one treatment in particular can cause horrendous constipation despite being one of the more effective treatments for HG symptoms. If a woman is prescribed ondansetron, then be sure to warn her of the signs of constipation. Advise her to seek help as soon as bowel movements become difficult. The last thing she needs is for it to get so bad she needs enemas and suffers painful evacuations.

Maintaining personal hygiene for HG sufferers can be tricky too as showering and brushing teeth can bring on violent emetic episodes. Ask her if she would like help and perhaps try to plan assistance with showering around an hour or so after her dose of anti-emetic, when they are most potent, if that is possible in the ward routine. It's an embarrassing and upsetting feeling knowing you haven't showered for weeks.

Potential Complications of HG

As with any patient suffering a serious illness there are a few other complications that can ensue and educating the woman to be aware of these can help in prevention.

Although not exhaustive, the following complications have been reported for women with HG and HCPs should be mindful of these when providing holistic care:

- Deep vein thrombosis (DVT), particular increased risk due to pregnancy, bed bound status and dehydration
- Pulmonary embolism, due to increased DVT risk
- Wernicke's encephalopathy, due to increased vomiting, prescribe thiamine (Vitamin B1) to combat risk and educate patient of the need for this supplement (many women mistakenly think this is an anti-emetic and when it is deemed not to help they stop taking it)
- Ante-natal depression, due to severity of symptoms and social isolation
- Pressure damage to tissue from bed-bound status and exacerbated by dehydration

If you are concerned a patient is depressed then referring her for counselling or to the peri-natal mental health team in your area is important. If these resources are limited then providing information about where else to seek help and support is useful. Further information is in the appendix.

There is information in chapter 6 for women to reduce the risk of DVT, PE and pressure damage and most wards carry written information for patients about these. If your ward is a maternity ward and doesn't have such information then a surgical or elderly ward will usually have a stock of leaflets.

Working in Partnership

Many women feel utterly out of control when they have HG and that's scary. By helping women to understand their condition better and self-manage in partnership with their HCPs, you give them back some control over their life and in turn help them to manage their condition. Listening to what does and doesn't work for each individual patient will help with making an effective treatment plan. Then ensuring that the woman understands which medication has been prescribed and why, and what the options are if those don't work, will hopefully increase compliance and help her feel a little more in control.

If she has been admitted for IV fluids, plan the discharge with her and she is less likely to come back in! If she would like to monitor her own fluid balance intake/output at home you could teach her how to do this as well as monitoring her own ketones. Using a care plan for self-monitoring symptoms at home and discussing with her how to know when she needs to come back in for more fluids or to step up medication means that admissions will hopefully be more appropriate and shorter in duration. Direct access to a ward is usually possible to arrange and in some areas, particularly increasingly in rural areas, IV fluids at home is possible to arrange for her. Women are currently able to receive IV at home in the South West of England and the Liverpool area and many more women are reporting their hospitals are offering day case IV rehydration. Birmingham Women's hospital are paving the way for day clinics and Sirona Care and Health in the Bath area are developing services for IV therapy at home, provided by Acute Care at Home nurses. They have a protocol in place and are currently developing a hyperemesis pathway. (see contacts in resources). Finally, call the woman's GP to ensure he/she is on board with the treatment plan.

Practical Tips for the Ward Environment

Sensory stimulation is a commonly reported trigger for sufferers. A woman suffering HG should ideally be in a side room, away from where food is served and noisy areas. Odours reported to particularly trigger symptoms include cigarette smoke, fatty foods, perfume and coffee. Most hospitals are now designated smoke-free areas, however in reality people do still smoke outside doorways and in car parks. If cigarette smoke is a particular trigger then being sensitive to this would be appreciated.

In a survey we conducted in 2014 of 345 women who had been admitted to hospital for hyperemesis in the last 5 years, 40% of them had encountered staff who had a strong smell of either cigarettes or perfume which made their condition worse. Therefore, although some hospital policies allow staff to wear 'light perfume' to work, in settings where hyperemesis sufferers could be encountered staff should be discouraged from wearing perfume. Unlike wearing modest make-up, perfume can aggravate a number of conditions from respiratory disorders to allergies, and both chemotherapy patients and pregnant women can be particularly sensitive to odours, however pleasant they may seem to others.

Ask for permission before discussing food and before mentioning food names in case it triggers nausea or vomiting (when you have vomited a particular food stuff enough times even the thought of it can trigger a powerful emetic response). Some women experience windows of nausea free time and enabling her to eat at these times is key.

Ensure a good stack of clean vomit bowls, and urine bowls if fluid balance is being monitored, are within easy reach at all times. Try to check regularly to remove used ones, or ask your health care assistant to prioritise this. Again this may sound so obvious to the excellent HCPs reading this, but from the survey mentioned above, of 345 women, 45% had to empty their own vomit or urine bowls while in hospital on at least one occasion. Sadly, we are even aware of women who found this particular indignity to be 'the final straw', and it directly contributed to their decision to terminate

The HG sufferer may be hard to cannulate due to dehydrated veins and extra care should be taken with this. Consider if an anaesthetic cream is an option, which it usually is if requested and time will allow.

Try to get the drugs to her on time. While we appreciate that it can tricky with busy drug rounds and constant interruptions, keeping blood levels stable with the anti-emetics is key to management. Perhaps any oral medications could be kept by the patient in a bedside locker so she can take them exactly when she needs them without relying on overstretched staff.

If possible, refer to a physiotherapist to minimise the effects of atrophy from prolonged bed rest. Measure her legs and prescribe TED stockings to reduce the risk of deep vein thrombosis.

Finally, Support Her.

HG can be a frustrating condition to manage for staff and sometimes the women may appear miserable and unwilling to help themselves. However the sufferer may be exhausted, scared, depressed and feeling guilty, stressed, and constantly nauseous. It's extremely difficult to do even the most simple tasks when feeling so overwhelmed with symptoms and emotions, and an inability to do things should not be confused with an unwillingness to do them. Many midwives and nurses I've (Caitlin) spoken to over the years express exacerbation at feeling like they can't help but actually, just being empathetic and supportive of a woman with HG can make the most incredible difference to her miserable experience. Studies have found women who felt well supported rated their physical and mental health more positively.

If you are concerned she is depressed, which is not a cause of HG but a common complication of it, (clearly 24/7 nausea and vomiting for weeks will make you depressed!), then refer for counselling or to the perinatal mental health team in your area if you have one. She may also be encouraged by a scan to see the baby, so it is worth finding out if that can be arranged.

You can also refer her to PSS for peer support from a registered and trained volunteer to reduce the isolation she may feel. The charity also has a forum she can go on to 'meet' other sufferers. Both PSS (UK) and The Hyperemesis Education and Research Foundation (USA) also have printable leaflets you can access. PSS can also send you an information pack with leaflets and posters for your clinic or ward. Consider having a supply that you can hand out to women and their partners and carers.

A Thorough Assessment of Nausea and Vomiting in Pregnancy and Hyperemesis Gravidarum

The assessment questions below and suggested investigations will help you ensure you are covering everything and give you the opportunity to answer the woman's questions and concerns. Without a thorough assessment, you can't go forward with developing a care plan, so taking the time to go through these questions is valuable. We have tried to keep them applicable to both the community and hospital setting as women with hyperemesis may present in a range of different settings. Due to this, some parts may be more or less relevant to your particular area of work. Our notes are in italics. We have used NVP rather than HG as a starting point as this is likely to be an assessment which will aid diagnosis of severity. However, if a woman has already been admitted with hyperemesis, then some sections will be less relevant.

General

- What stage of pregnancy from last monthly period (LMP) are you?
- Is this your first pregnancy?
- Did you experience nausea and vomiting of pregnancy (NVP) in previous pregnancy?
- If yes, was the NVP/HG better or worse than this pregnancy?
- How long ago did the NVP start, from LMP?
  NVP usually starts about day 39 (5.5 weeks) from LMP. In about 13% of pregnant women, NVP will start before a missed period, and for 90% of women, NVP will start before day 56 from LMP.

Vomiting

- Are you vomiting?
- If yes, how long ago did vomiting start?
- How many times a day are you vomiting?
- Is vomiting getting more frequent?
- How much fluid are you vomiting each time –
  i.e. a cupful or a) more b) less?
- Have you been vomiting blood or bile?

Signs of Dehydration

- Have you got a dry mouth and lips?
- Is your urine very dark or of small quantity which you pass less frequently than 8 hourly?
- Does your urine contain ketones?
  (Ketostix tests are available from a chemist or online about £6 for a container of 50). 3 or 4+ of ketones is a factor for immediate

admission to hospital but any ketones should be considered for admission. Some women will know what ketones are, particularly if they have suffered HG before, whereas women in their first pregnancies likely will not.

Weight Loss

- Have you lost weight compared to your pre-pregnancy weight? If so, how much?
  Loss greater than 5% of pre-pregnancy weight is significant and is one factor to be considered for hospital admission.

Nausea

- Do you have episodes of nausea?
- Or, is the nausea constant?
- If episodic, then do you keep a daily diary of your episodes so that you can judge when you will be able to eat and drink and be ready to do so?
- If the nausea is constant, then is it affecting your ability to eat and/or drink?
- Does anything make your NVP worse?
  Usual replies include noxious odours, fried or fatty food, cooked food, meat or fish, tea or coffee, smell of perfume, cigarette smoke, being hungry, positional change, movement, fatigue, and others.
- Does travelling make your NVP worse?
  If distance to a hospital is a problem then consider if home IV is possible in their area.
- Does anything improve your NVP?
  Evidence-based advice includes the following points, but remember that for full-blown hyperemesis, eating and drinking at all may be impossible.

1. ***Eating and drinking.*** *Eat what you like (according to current government guidelines for pregnancy), when you like, including your cravings, in small frequent quantities and when you first wake up, to prevent feeling too hungry. Drink what you like (according to current government guidelines for pregnancy). Try lemonade, cold water, sucking ice cubes, or sorbets.*
2. ***Rest.*** *Women say rest is the second most important way to relieve their*

NVP. Lying down when NVP is severe and after eating a meal is often effective. You will not be able to 'work off' NVP by taking increased exercise.

3. ***Avoid unpleasant odours.** Your nose is your worst enemy at present, and odours which may normally have been no problem may now make your nausea much worse. You may smell odours no one else can detect.*
4. ***Support.** Get help if possible, with household duties, shopping, and with your children.*
5. ***Avoid** loud noises, bright lights, and other sensory stimulation.*
6. ***Enjoy** what you really like, for example, music, TV, DVDs, radio, reading, or whatever you can manage.*

Effects on Well-being and Lifestyle

- Does NVP affect your Activities of Daily Living (ADLs), that is, shopping, cooking, housework, parenting?
  As soon as a woman's ADLs are affected, this indicates that safe effective medication, usually tablets, is advisable to treat NVP. Early treatment reduces the incidence of admission to hospital for HG.
- Does NVP affect your mood or attitude to life, for example, does it make you feel depressed?
  50% of women with severe NVP feel depressed most of the time due to the condition.
- Does your NVP affect your partner's lifestyle or employment?
  There is on line support and information for partners, and there is a section in this book for them.
- Do you have paid employment? If yes, are you allowed to take things easy at work or have time off?
  Up-to-date information about employment rights is on the PSS website.

Treatment

- Are you taking a pregnancy vitamin with folic acid?
- Have you taken any complimentary or alternative treatments for nausea for NVP, for example, herbal treatment, ginger, anything from a health

food shop, or used acupressure bands? If yes, what was it, and was it helpful?
Asking what they have tried is very different to suggesting that they try these things. Knowing what they have already tried will aid your assessment and help them feel listened to. It is also an opportunity to discuss evidence-based treatment and risk/benefit assessments.

- How do you feel about taking tablets to treat your NVP if you were sure they would not affect your baby?
Here, you can reassure that there is safe effective treatment for NVP.

- Have you been prescribed any treatment by your GP or by hospital doctors? If so, then what?

- Is there anything you would like to ask us about NVP?
Be careful not to give false promises of complete recovery at 12 weeks. It is better to be realistic about the duration of hyperemesis and discuss longer-term coping strategies for the next few months. Disappointment over the pregnancy will already be profoundly felt, so a 'prepare for the worst, hope for the best' attitude can be helpful.

Future Support

- What support do you have at home?
- What form of future support do you need to help manage your condition?
- Would you like a referral to the charity Pregnancy Sickness Support?

Investigations

The following investigations should be standard during the diagnosis and management of the patient with hyperemesis although ongoing frequency will depend on the case severity and the initial results:

- Weight of patient
- Urinalysis
- Full blood count (FBC), urea and electrolytes (U&E) – possibly daily
- Liver function test (LFT), thyroid function test (TFT)
- Calcium and phosphate levels if severe

- Blood glucose
- Mid stream specimen urine (MSSU)

A MUST (Malnutrition Universal Screening Tool) or PUQE (Pregnancy-Unique Quantification of Emesis) should be used to assess the effectiveness of intervention. The PUQE tool is available in the Appendix.

On a first admission, a scan may be appropriate to assess for multiple foetuses and rule out a molar pregnancy.

Developing a Care Plan

One day, we hope that a solid, standard, evidence-based care plan for any woman admitted with hyperemesis will be automatically initiated regardless of where in the country they are suffering. But until that day, we need HCPs to be making their own care plans and they will have to be based on the evidence we have to date combined with common sense. All qualified nurses and midwives should be experienced in writing a care plan as it makes up the foundation of the care they and their colleagues provide to their patients.

Women who are trying for a subsequent pregnancy after a previous hyperemesis pregnancy should be encouraged to develop a care plan in advance, and a sample of this plan is available in the chapter 'Preparation for the Hyperemesis Pregnancy'.

However, for women in their first hyperemesis pregnancy who have just been diagnosed or admitted with hyperemesis, this is a sample care plan for the ward environment.

Care Plan for the Patient Suffering with Hyperemesis Gravidarum

Care Plan for ....

Date of admission ....

Weeks gestation at admission ....

Pregnancy number ....

Children at home ....

History of twins: yes / no ....

Weight at admission:.. KG

Height .... CM

BMI ....

Patient reported weight loss.. or

% of pre-pregnancy weight loss ....

Blood Pressure ..../.....................

Ketone level on admission ....

TED Stockings provided? YES / NO ....

Aims of Care Plan:

1. Reduce nausea and vomiting
2. Reduce presence of ketones and increase hydration
3. Prevent further weight loss
4. Provide emotional and psychosocial support to...
5. Provide a comfortable environment for...

Nursing Actions for Care Plan:

1. Reduce Nausea and Vomiting

- Ensure medication is provided on time to enable stable blood levels of anti-emetics.
- Reduce sensory stimulation by providing a side room away from 'smelly areas', if possible, and ensuring staff are quiet and free from perfume whilst providing care.
- Provide snacks when required where possible.
- Review effectiveness of medication and interventions daily or as required, using MUST or PUQE tool.

2. Reduce Presence of Ketones

- Provide IV fluids as per prescription. *(See Part 2, Chapter 5 for more info)*
- Warm IV fluids to 37 degrees before administration, if possible. *This is to reduce calorific loss from cold IV fluid administration.*
- Encourage oral fluids when they can be tolerated.
- Provide information on suitable fluids for pregnancy and tips on getting fluids, for example, via ice lollies.
- Monitor ketones as per hospital policy or three times per day.

3. Prevent Further Weight Loss

- Encourage oral food intake where possible.
- Provide information on fortifying food and fluid. *(Information available on PSS website and in chapter 6)*
- Ensure medication regime is controlling vomiting and nutrient loss. Adjust timings to maximise ability to eat at mealtimes.
- Provide snacks as and when .... feels able to eat.

4. Provide Emotional and Psychosocial Support to

....

- Where available, discuss referral to peri-natal mental health team for sup port with psychological impact of HG and refer if appropriate.
- Provide information about PSS charity and make referral to support net work if required.
- Ensure .... has an advocate for ward rounds with doctors if she is struggling with speaking due to nausea and vomiting.
- Ensure informed consent is obtained for treatments.
- Provide written information about hyperemesis and any treatments or medication.

5. Provide a Comfortable Environment for.......................................

- Provide a side room where possible to reduce sensory stimulation such as smell and sound and reduce distress from public vomiting and episodes of incontinence.
- Ensure staff are free from perfumes or cigarette smoke.
- Provide pressure relieving mattress to reduce the risk of pressure damage from prolonged bed rest.
- Ensure vomit bowls and urine samples are removed promptly and ad equate empty receptacles provided.

For a Medication Management Plan, please see the next chapter.

CHAPTER 4

Management, Treatments, and Medications

When it comes to treating severe NVP and HG, you will most likely find a million different opinions but very little evidence. A lot of this is due to the lack of accessible information both on the nature of severe NVP and HG and the safety of certain medications. Yet information does exist, and it is our hope that within this chapter, you will find all you need to make an informed choice about your treatment options and develop the ability to advocate for yourself.

> *One of the overwhelming memories of my pregnancy was the feeling that nobody believed I should be taking medication. As I didn't have the energy to research it myself, it took me many weeks and multiple appointments with various GPs to finally be prescribed an anti-emetic that helped. I was refused IV hydration, only now realising how desperately I needed it, and I found that even when medication was finally prescribed, everybody and his dog seemed to have an opinion on why I shouldn't be 'risking my baby' like that.*

(Amanda Shortman, Author)

Amanda's experience is far from unique in this respect and so we want to state right now: There are several anti-emetic medications that are considered safe for use during pregnancy. Most of these have been used for many years without any evidence of teratogenic effect on the foetus, and there is research available that indicates as much. There is, of course, scope for far more research into these particular medications, but research does exist which can help you and your healthcare provider decide on the best treatment for you.

Furthermore, this list is not exhaustive, and there are more and more drugs coming onto the market and being used in pregnancy. As more and more women used them, data about their safety and efficiency will increase. If you have been prescribed a medication not mentioned in this book and are worried or concerned then speak to your doctor about the evidence base for it or contact the Charities listed in Appendix 1. With the exception of trials, for which consent will be specifically gained, for a doctor to prescribe a medication they will already be confident in the safety of the drug's use in pregnancy and should be happy to discuss it.

If there are safe treatment options, why can it be so hard to find a doctor who is willing to prescribe anti-emetic medications?

The problem with prescribing medications for pregnant women comes from the fact that no drug is licensed for use during pregnancy in the United Kingdom. Many doctors are reluctant to prescribe anything for fear that something may happen to the foetus and the medication may be blamed. The issue here may well lie in the fact that 1–3% of all live births will involve a major birth defect of some kind. This is a natural occurrence, but if an unlicensed drug has been administered, the prescribing doctor would potentially need to prove that the birth defect was not caused by the medication.

That is not to say that the medications cause birth defects. There are plenty of studies that show no rise in the percentage of birth defects naturally occurring following the use of various anti-emetic drugs. But without the backing of a license for use in pregnancy, the onus falls on the prescribing doctor. And if that doctor is unaware of the treatment options available for severe NVP and HG and the safety data connected to them, then the patient has a hard battle to get appropriate treatment.

Of course, this is further complicated by the fact that the majority of us have no medical background and therefore no knowledge of the treatment options ourselves. We are likely to take what our doctors tells us as 'gospel' and listen to all those who tell us that taking medications during pregnancy is unwise, dangerous, or even selfish. Too many people refer automatically to the effects of Thalidomide which, though extremely serious, are not relevant to the treatment options offered today. Since the use of Thalidomide resulted in such pronounced birth defects, there has been much more emphasis on researching the potential teratogenic effects of any medication that might be prescribed during pregnancy. As such, various anti-emetics are available today which have been used for decades without any such concerns and to suffer needlessly due to concerns over this is an avoidable experience if you have the relevant information.

Understanding the term "risk"

It can be scary for women when doctors talk about risks, particularly when they mention things like cleft palate or heart defects. Headlines in newspapers can add to fear-mongering when they talk about certain medications "doubling risks" for the baby without accurate explanation. This can be worrying for women who are already taking the medications mentioned in order to maintain the pregnancy. You may even be faced with friends or relatives coming to you with articles and internet posts claiming various scary risks.

Let's use a hypothetical example to get "risk" in perspective. Suppose the base line rate for heart defects is one in 1,000. That means that even in normal, healthy pregnancies one baby in every 1,000 will be born with a defect in their heart. Now supposing you are at a point where you are so seriously ill that you need to take strong medication for hyperemesis gravidarum or you are at risk of various complications for your own health and the baby's, if you don't take the medication you may have little option but to terminate this baby you really want. You agree to take the treatment but then read that the treatment you are on may possibly double the risk of cardiac defects. That can sound very scary and dramatic but it actually means that the baby now has a one in 500 chance of a cardiac defect instead of one in 1,000 (or you could say it has a 2 in 1,000 chance). On top of that you need to factor in the risk chronic dehydration and malnutrition poses to the foetus. There are less studies looking at the effect of not treating HG and it's less "news-worthy" in today's culture.

We are by no means saying that you should take a drug which "doubles" the risk of cardiac defects. Rather we are trying to help you understand what that statistic means for you to weigh up your choices and help you make decisions. And in the days of sensationalist news stories particularly when it comes to pregnancy we hope this explanation will help you assess articles and research you may read during your pregnancy and give you a way of explaining it to concerned relatives.

I am still concerned about taking anti-emetic medications? Do I have to take them?

The simple answer to this is no. You never have to take anything that you feel uncomfortable with and should always be given the information you need to make an informed choice over your treatment.

If you feel that you would rather continue without medication, then please do skip to the following chapters which focus on coping strategies and the emotional impact of severe NVP and HG. However, if you feel that you need and want some treatment but are still a little unsure of the options, then we hope that the rest of this chapter will help alleviate some of those concerns.

The Importance of Treating Severe Nausea and Vomiting in Pregnancy and Hyperemesis

When left untreated, severe nausea and/or vomiting can lead to dehydration, the production of ketones (when your body starts to break down fat instead of glucose due to a lack of sufficient nutritional intake), rapid weight loss, electrolyte imbalances, and, in more severe cases, can even begin to damage the internal organs through the stress on the body. Therefore, the aim of treatment is always to try and limit the symptoms that lead to such effects (i.e., try and reduce the level of nausea and frequency of vomiting so that the patient can adequately hydrate herself and begin to eat more).

When a woman becomes dehydrated during pregnancy, it is possible to refer her to hospital for IV hydration. Often this is the point at which a woman is diagnosed with HG or when anti-emetic drugs are first prescribed. However, IV hydration alone may not be enough to keep symptoms at bay, and some women find that they have multiple readmissions once they have returned home and their symptoms of nausea and/or vomiting prevent them from adequately hydrating themselves. For others, an admission to hospital may never be suggested despite a constant battle with dehydration.

It is interesting to note that there used to be a licensed drug called Bendectin that was prescribed for pregnant women suffering from severe NVP and HG in various countries including the United Kingdom. However, due to claims around the safety of the drug (all of which were later found to be unfounded), the drug was removed from the market. Following this, the rate of hospital admissions due to severe sickness during pregnancy doubled over 5 years. However, a similar drug named Diclectin is currently licensed for use during pregnancy in Canada, and since its introduction, the rate of hospital admissions in Canada has dropped dramatically, a trend not seen in other countries where anti-emetic drugs remain unlicensed during pregnancy.

So, it is clear that anti-emetic drugs can play a huge part in reducing the severity of symptoms a woman with severe NVP or hyperemesis experiences and enable her to better manage these symptoms. But still the issue remains that many healthcare providers are unaware of or reluctant to prescribe these during pregnancy, and as such women feel worried or guilty about taking them. So let's look at some studies that focus on the safety of anti-emetic drug use during pregnancy.

A summary of the Medications Currently in Use

Please note that the field of medicine is constantly changing and that between writing this book, publishing it, and you reading it, the research about the individual medications may have changed. New research is constantly being carried out, and safety data is constantly emerging. For the most recent information regarding medications, please contact Pregnancy Sickness Support.

Pyridoxone, Vitamin B6

Pyridoxone is vitamin B6 which is required to maintain a healthy nervous system. It has been shown to be effective in helping NVP in two randomised controlled trials against placebo (one trial at 30 mgs/daily, the other at 75 mgs/daily). A retrospective cohort study concluded that pyridoxine monotherapy had no increased risk for major malformations. There are no apparent side effects.

Current research supports a dose of 10 mg 1 tablet four times per day (although much higher doses are used in Canada). These are available over the counter and are suggested as a pre-emptive measure for sufferers planning subsequent pregnancies.

Antihistamines

Old-fashioned H1 receptor antagonist anti-histamines such as cyclizine (brand name Valoid) and promethazine (brand name Avomine) should be used as a first-line treatment. If started early, they can prevent a deterioration of symptoms and possibly prevent moderate to severe NVP becoming HG.

There is plenty of evidence suggesting that these antihistamines have no human teratogenic potential (teratogenic means harmful defects in the foetus). Pooled data from seven randomised controlled trials demonstrate that these antihistamines are effective in the treatment of NVP.

Drowsiness is a common side effect of these medications and should not be taken without medical advice, although they are available over the counter. It can take a couple of weeks to become accustomed to the drowsy effect.

Cyclizine given via IV in hospital can be quite an unpleasant experience for many women. It can sting as it's administered and cause dizziness.

The above combined make up the components of the licensed Canadian drug Diclectin (Diclegis in the USA). They are generally the first step in treatment in the United Kingdom, and further medication can be added as required.

Thiamine (Vitamin B1)

This is often prescribed as part of hospital protocol because excessive vomiting can lead to a deficiency in vitamin B1 (thiamine), which can cause a condition called Wernicke's encephalopathy. This condition can be fatal but is prevented by replacing the thiamine B1. If you are vomiting excessively, you need to attempt to take this important supplement when you can.

Metoclopramide (Brand Name Maxalon)

There is limited information on its safety in pregnancy, although what has been published is reassuring and it has been used in pregnancy for many years now. There are a very limited number of studies that indicate the effectiveness of metoclopramide in the treatment of NVP. Side effects include drowsiness, restlessness, and occasionally extra pyramidal effects (such as tremor, slurred speech, anxiety, distress, and others). This is a prescription-only medication.

It is used more commonly in America where the brand name is Reglan; the Food and Drug Administration (FDA) in America has recently recommended that it can be used for up to 12 weeks, but after this, side effects can become more severe. However, recent European guidance states that metoclopramide should only be used for up to 5 days to prevent adverse neurological side effects. For that reason, women in the United Kingdom may find that they are prescribed this only to have treatment stopped after 5 days. Other women may find that they tolerate it well and their doctor keeps prescribing it despite the guidance. Discuss any concerns about this treatment with your doctor. Bear in mind that the guidance to stop after 5 days is not due to a potential risk to the foetus but due to side effects for the mother. Report any side effects to your doctor.

Women may also find the side effects less tolerable when given via IV and in doses over 40 mg per day side effects are more common and/or severe, so should be avoided.

Prochlorperazine

Prochlorperazine (brand name Stemetil) is one of a number of drugs called phenothiazine. Prospective and retrospective cohort studies, case-control, and record linkage studies of patients with exposure to various and multiple phenothiazines have not found an increased risk of malformations in the infant. Three randomised controlled trials in severe NVP found it to be effective for controlling symptoms. Side effects, much like metoclopramide, include drowsiness, restlessness, and occasional extra pyramidal effects (such as tremor, slurred speech, anxiety, distress, and others). These are prescription-only medications, and if you experience any side effects, discuss them with your doctor.

Domperidone

Domperidone (brand name Motilium) works in two ways. First, by speeding up the passage of food through the stomach into the intestine, this in turn prevents nausea and vomiting. It also prevents food from flowing the wrong way through the stomach and so can help with reflux. Second, domperidone blocks dopamine receptors found in an area of the brain known as the chemoreceptor trigger zone (CTZ). The CTZ is activated by nerve messages from the stomach when an irritant is present or when certain chemicals are in the blood stream, such as pregnancy hormones. Once activated, messages are sent to the vomiting centre which sends messages to the gut and triggers vomiting. By blocking the dopamine receptors in the CTZ, domperidone prevents nausea messages from being sent to the vomiting centre and in turn reduces the nausea and vomiting.

As with many of the treatments mentioned here, the safety of domperidone has not been established in proper medical trials. However, it has been used for a number of years in pregnancy and as yet no adverse effect on the foetus has been found.

Domperidone can be given as a suppository (in your back passage) which some women may find easier then swallowing orally.

Because it works in a very different way to the other treatments, it can be particularly effective in combination with other medications. Less side effects tend to be reported with domperidone.

Ondansetron

If you've already been on Facebook or had a browse around the Internet, you'll likely have heard about ondansetron, or Zofran, the brand name. It is a relatively new medication which was originally used to treat nausea and vomiting caused by chemotherapy for cancer patients but is increasingly used for HG.

Research regarding the safety of this drug is increasing. A study in Canada by the Motherisk program looked at foetal outcomes for mothers who had taken ondansetron as well as mothers who had taken other anti-emetics and compared them to the baseline rate of birth defects. It was found that there was no increase in the rate of birth defects for mothers who had taken ondansetron.

A more recent study in Denmark by Pasternak et al. (2013) looked at 1,233 women exposed to ondansetron between weeks 7 and 12 of pregnancy (from LMP) and compared the birth defect rate with that of 4,932 women not exposed to ondansetron. They found that the birth defect rate was 2.9%, at birth, for both groups. A literature review by PSS found the baseline risk of 1–3% for a major congenital birth defect at birth for all pregnancies which is in line with this research. This is very encouraging research, but as with all these medications, more research is needed.

It can be taken orally, as an injection, as a suppository (inside your rectum) or as an 'oro-dispersal' tablet (melted on the tongue), which is particularly useful for a lot of women.

It is a prescription-only medication, and side effects include severe constipation and headaches. In 2012, a side effect of QT elevation (a heart arrhythmia which can be very dangerous) was found in patients receiving doses of 32 mg IV in one go. As a result of this, the US Food and Drug Administration (FDA) issued a 'black box warning' for ondansetron in America. However, this is only for very high single doses, IV, and it is highly unlikely pregnant women in the United Kingdom would ever be prescribed such a dose. At the time of writing, the standard 16 mg in 24 hours is still considered safe for the mother and has not been found to have any adverse cardiac effects. Your doctor may wish to take an electrocardiogram (ECG) before giving ondansetron though, and if you have a history of heart problems, you may not be offered this medication.

Unfortunately, despite its efficiency for controlling NVP symptoms, many women report to the authors that the constipation side effect of ondansetron is so profound and painful that they cannot tolerate the treatment at all. Advice about constipation should be given at the time of prescribing along with information about seeking further help if this becomes a problem.

Steroids

There is increasing evidence for the use of steroids for the treatment of the more severe end of the nausea and vomiting spectrum, known as HG. Steroids have been used for a number of years in pregnancy for conditions such as acute asthma and Crohn's disease. There may be a small increased risk of oral clefting associated with the use of corticosteroids and many authorities say that they should not be used to treat NVP in the first 12 weeks of pregnancy; however, more recent studies are questioning this. Many doctors are now happy to use steroids after 8 weeks gestation (10 weeks from LMP), and the authors know of women who have used them as early as 6 weeks in very severe cases. The data is really increasing for the effectiveness of corticosteroids to treat severe HG.

Corticosteroids need to be given under medical supervision and assessment. They are normally started in hospital intravenously at a high dose and then tapered off over a number of weeks orally at home.

If your hyperemesis is so severe that you are considering termination of the pregnancy, then your doctor should be willing to try steroids first.

Suggested doses for steroid therapy are (Taylor, 2009) as follows:

- Prednisolone, oral 10 mg 3 times daily (tdi), increasing to 15 mg tdi and 20 mg tdi until vomiting is controlled.

  OR, if oral treatment is not tolerated

- Hydrocortisone IV 50 mg tdi, increasing to 75 mg tdi and 100 mg tdi until vomiting is controlled. Switch to oral prednisolone once fluids are tolerated.

Antacids

Ranitidine is a histamine-2 (H2) receptor antagonist and works in a way that reduces the amount of gastric acid produced by H2 receptor cells in the stomach. It works quickly, but the effect doesn't last as long, so regular doses are required. Omeprozole is a proton pump inhibitor, and it reduces gastric acid production by inhibiting the enzyme system (proton pump) in the gastric parietal cell. It takes longer to work, but the effect lasts longer and generally one a day dose is required, although the effects may last up to 3 days.

There has been limited research into the efficiency and safety of acid and reflux suppressing medications. But what research there has been is very encouraging and suggests they do not have a teratogenic effect if taken during pregnancy and are safe even in the first trimester. In terms of efficiency, there is certainly an increasing realisation that combining acid and reflux suppressants with anti-emetics can aid in controlling HG symptoms, which are exacerbated by acid reflux. Not just the actual vomiting but the pain experienced when vomiting acidic liquid and the gastric irritation and potential damage to the oesophagus may be helped by antacid medications. It has been suggested that the 'third trimester relapse' which is commonly reported to be experienced by HG sufferers can be reduced with these treatments although as yet there is little research to support the claim.

The Motherisk programme in Canada advocates these medications as standard for women with moderate to severe pregnancy sickness as part of a holistic treatment regime. The experiences of the authors from working with women with HG is that these medications are very helpful in the treatment of HG and women gain huge benefit from having one of these combined into their treatment plan. Their use in the United Kingdom is currently undervalued in HG management.

OTHER THERAPIES

Intravenous Fluids

Intravenous (IV, meaning directly into the vein) fluids are given to correct dehydration, and medication can be given through the IV port when oral medication is unable to be tolerated.

Although IV therapy is common and some doctors would prefer to repeatedly prescribe IV fluids rather than medication for pregnant women, they are not without risk. The main risk associated with IV therapy lies at the site of cannulation. Blood and fluids can leak in to surrounding tissues causing damage and pain. Repeated cannulations can lead to destruction of the vein by scar tissue making future cannulations impossible. Infection is a big risk, and in the days of antibiotic-resistant strains of bacteria such as MRSA, treating infection can be difficult.

However, IV fluid replacement does remain an effective treatment for dehydration, which actually can cause nausea and vomiting. Women often feel temporary but effective relief from a few bags of IV fluids.

Recently, in the United Kingdom, there is an increasing service provision for IV fluids to be administered at home which is an exciting development for HG sufferers who can find the trip to and from hospital and the ward environment quite distressing and exacerbating of symptoms. In particular, a pioneering service led by community nurse Emma Moxham, near Bath in the south west of England, has been successfully providing IV at home for women with HG for about 3 years now and interest in the service is increasing in other areas too. They have developed a care pathway for the service and their details are in the appendix should you wish to find out more.

Dr Marjory Maclean, consultant obstetrician at Ayrshire Maternity Unit in Scotland, suggests a suitable regime for fluid replacement as follows:

Fluid Replacement

- If significant ketonuria, 1000 ml 0.9% sodium chloride intravenously over 2 to 4 hours. Hartmann's can also be used.
- Thereafter fluids should be reduced to 500 ml 4–6 hourly, the regime being guided by U&E results, which should be performed daily, particularly for monitoring potassium levels.
- Avoid glucose initially as it contains insufficient sodium and especially as Wernicke's encephalopathy may be precipitated unless thiamine is given first.

Total Parental Nutrition

Total Parental Nutrition (TPN) is a 'complete feed' delivered IV (if short term) or via a Peripherally Inserted Central Catheter (PICC) or Central Catheter (if treatment will go on for more than 2 weeks). It is far more commonly used in America but is still pretty rare in the United Kingdom. It can sound like a good solution for women at their worst point, but it is not without significant risk. If your doctor feels this is the way forward for you, then you are unlikely to have much choice as it is not a treatment which is embarked upon lightly. If your doctor does not want to go down this route yet but you would like it discussed as an option, then try to discuss it with them, but be aware of the potential risks and side effects. These include but are not limited to

1. Infection. TPN for any length of time is given through a PICC or central line, which is like an IV but it goes centrally to your heart, see the glossary for further explanation. An infection in a PICC line is far more serious than an infection in a normal IV catheter. An infection in a PICC line can be fatal.
2. Long-term IV lines or PICC lines have a higher risk of blood clots forming and these can be fatal also.
3. The insertion of the long-term catheter or PICC lines carries risks of pneumothorax, accidental arterial puncture, and catheter-related sepsis.
4. If TPN is replacing oral intake completely, then bile stasis in the gall balder can ensue rapidly due to the lack of use of the digestive system. Although this is reversible, it should not be underestimated, particularly for long-term use of TPN.
5. Refeeding syndrome. When the body has been starved for more than about 5 days, the reintroduction of food can cause serious metabolic disturbances. This is not just a complication of TPN but of HG generally and is one of the reasons women are commonly prescribed thiamine (vitamin B1) in hospital for HG.

Enteral Nutrition

This is a liquid feed given either via a Nasogastric Tube (NG tube) or a Percutaneous Endoscopic Gastrostomy (PEG). See the glossary for further detail but brief explanations of these:

- An NG tube is a long tube that goes in through the nose, down the back of the throat and into the stomach or jejunum

- The PEG is inserted during a surgical procedure to implant it through the abdomen into the stomach. Sometimes, the tube will go further down into the jejunum which is often tolerated better. Surgical procedures during pregnancy carry further risks, and this is rarely done in the United Kingdom.

Both procedures are pretty unpleasant, and in the United Kingdom, it would be very rare for an HG sufferer to be given a PEG. Enteral feeding is however much safer than TPN, and your doctor may want to see if you tolerate an NG tube before considering TPN. Unfortunately, the nature of HG means that women often do not tolerate NG tubes very well and could be at higher risk of complications such as tube displacement from vomiting and lung aspiration from a displaced tube. Because women with HG often have a highly sensitive gag reflex, slowed gastric emptying, reflux, and frequent vomiting, the risks of dislodging the tube is higher. Also women may find the smell of the liquid feed a trigger for vomiting.

Risks of refeeding syndrome are also present with enteral feeding, as with TPN, and this should be closely monitored.

Termination

Whether termination is a 'treatment' is debatable, it certainly cures the symptoms at the time. Many women who experience HG, at some point in their pregnancy will consider termination as an option. The Hyperemesis Education and Research Foundation in America found that over 10% of pregnancies complicated by HG were terminated. More often than not, this is due to inadequate treatment of symptoms and a lack of support and understanding from HCPs, employers, and the general public. A large survey by PSS in 2013 found the termination rate in United Kingdom to be 9%, and of them, only 7% had been given steroids and 20% had been given ondansetron. That is a truly depressing state of affairs!

If you are considering or have recently terminated due to HG, then please see chapter 9 on Termination.

Complementary and Alternative Medicine and Non-Medical Intervention

Pregnancy is a state of being which seems to be absolutely rife with pseudoscience and opportunity for spending money. It is also a time when you will be particularly targeted by complementary and alternative medicine (CAM) therapies claiming to be able to cure any and every pregnancy discomfort and ailment. Whether or not CAM has a place in the modern world is too big a topic for discussion on these pages; indeed, there are plenty of books on the subject available.

A survey conducted by Dr O'Hara found that there was a very high (99%) awareness of the various CAM treatments available for pregnancy sickness such as ginger, acupressure, acupuncture, homoeopathy, and so on.

However, as you are very likely to come across people (probably on a daily basis), including family, friends, work colleagues, complete strangers, and your HCPs, who will all suggest a whole host of CAM treatments from the plausible to the absurd, we thought it best to include a summary of the options.

This is where the distinction between normal pregnancy sickness and severe NVP/HG is needed. The chances that are if you are reading this book, you are at the moderate to severe end of the pregnancy sickness spectrum and therefore the chances of a CAM helping your symptoms is highly unlikely – if only it were that simple! That's not to say that CAM treatments won't help at all. For women with normal or mild pregnancy sickness, they may help significantly, even if it is with a placebo effect. Even for women with severe NVP or HG, they may give a little comfort from symptoms and provide psychological support, knowing that you are 'trying everything'. Bear in mind though that many CAM therapies were around long before modern medicine, back in the days when women died from HG. It is the modern treatments that have reduced the deaths and so we feel it important to note here that any CAM therapies you try should not be seen as an alternative to the treatments offered by your healthcare provider but rather as an addition to them.

So what do we know about the CAM options?

Acupressure Bands: Stimulation of the P6 point, located three fingers breadth above the wrist, has been used for many years to treat nausea from a variety of causes. Trials of a non-blinded randomised nature (i.e. the placebo effect could influence the results) have shown a decrease of persisting nausea by at least 50%. Bands worn at the wrist (e.g. travel sickness or 'morning sickness' bands) that apply pressure may be a simple way of stimulating the P6 point. There are no theoretical concerns about the safety of acupressure in pregnancy.

Authors' note by Caitlin: Although the manufactures of acupressure bands don't mention side effects of long-term use, please be aware that using them continuously for 9 months can lead to pressure damage and scarring on your wrists.

Ginger: Six randomised controlled trials with a total of 675 participants were conducted and found that ginger extract at 1000 mgs per day may be an effective treatment for NVP. However, the small number of patients in each of these studies allocated to receive ginger (n = 303) may have been insufficient to properly test the safety of ginger with regards to pregnancy outcome. Ginger is a non-regulated food product, and most preparations available are of variable purity and composition, so dose is uncertain. Side effects include heartburn and thromboxane synthetase inhibition, that is, inhibits platelet aggregation. Caution should be exercised while taking very high doses of ginger. Sufferers also report to the authors that ginger is a painful substance to vomit.

Others: Some women seem to find help through hypnotherapy and acupuncture treatments. A few women claim to have had the illness 'stopped in its tracks' by acupuncture, but success varies between individual patients and it tends to be expensive. The impact of the placebo effect should also be accounted for and the experience of having a professional 'taking care' of you and helping with relaxation for the duration of a session can also help. These remedies are worth a try if you can afford it but have a back-up plan in case it doesn't work. They can also help psychologically as you will likely be asked constantly if you've tried them – being able to say that you have can be positive.

It is also worth bearing in mind that many CAM treatments are 'real' in that they have an effect on the body, that is, taking ginger or inserting needles into the skin (acupuncture). Therefore, if you are nervous about taking prescribed medication because they aren't licensed for pregnancy (but have vast amounts of data regarding their use), then the same logic should apply to CAM therapies. They should have sufficient research providing evidence of their safety in pregnancy for both mother and foetus before you try them, and the practitioner should be registered with a reputable organisation which insists on professional practices such as ongoing training, continual monitoring of practice, and up-to-date insurance. Just because they are considered 'natural' doesn't mean they are safe, rather safety needs to be proven by research, regardless of efficiency.

Research addressing the safety of anti-emetic medications

Use of anti-emetic drugs during pregnancy in Sweden, By Asker, Norstedt Wikner and Källén, 2005

Though this study was conducted in Sweden, many of the anti-emetic drugs prescribed are the same that women are prescribed here in the United Kingdom. These include cyclizine, metoclopramide, ondansetron, Prochlorperazine and promethazine.

Information was collated from the Swedish Medical Birth Register during the period from 1 July 1995 to 2002. Women who reported the use of anti-emetics were compared with all women who gave birth during the study period. This allowed the researchers to not only understand the use of anti-emetics during pregnancy but also compare the delivery outcomes of those women prescribed anti-emetic drugs with those who weren't.

During the study period, 29,804 women (which totalled 4.5% of all women studied) gave birth to 31,130 infants following the use of anti-emetics during pregnancy. Interestingly, 23,396 (78% of all those prescribed anti-emetics) reported the use of anti-emetic drugs at their first antenatal appointment (usually held between weeks 10 and 12) without any further mention of these at later appointments. This suggests that a large percentage of women who took anti-emetics during their first trimester may have discontinued them later on.

A total of 4,018 (13%) reported no anti-emetic drugs at their initial appointment but were prescribed them later in pregnancy, and 2,394 (8%) reported use both early in pregnancy and at a later date. What this study also shows is that the large majority of women who were prescribed anti-emetic drugs started taking them within the first trimester.

The study looks at many more factors and is well worth a read if you are interested in studying this in more detail. However, as we are currently interested in the safety of anti-emetics, we shall keep this as simple as possible.

The study compared the rate of congenital malformations (birth defects) in babies born to women who had used anti-emetic drugs with those who hadn't. Some minor malformations, such as an unstable hip, were not uniformly recorded in the register and so were removed from the analysis. This left 684 (2.2%) of infants born to women who had used anti-emetic drugs compared to 2.5% of women who had not taken anti-emetic drugs.

This led the study's authors to state that they, 'found no signs that the drugs had a teratogenic effect, but for some of the drugs studied the numbers of exposures was low' (i.e. some of the anti-emetics were not prescribed as frequently as others).

The authors also state, however, that, 'antiemetic therapy does not usually begin during thc most sensitive part of organ formation, and we were unable to identify women who had used antiemetic drugs very early in their pregnancy'. By this, they mean that although a large majority of women reported use of anti-emetics at around 10–12 weeks during their first antenatal appointment, there is no data to show at which point prior to that they had begun taking the medication and therefore it is impossible for them to say categorically that anti-emetics are safe for use in the very early weeks of pregnancy.

Although this study cannot provide adequate evidence of the safety of anti-emetics during the very earliest weeks of pregnancy, there is increasing research regarding the safety of early treatment. During your first pregnancy, it can be a struggle to get treatment straight away, but there is increasingly strong evidence for the benefit of taking pre-emptive medication during subsequent pregnancies (which is discussed further in chapter 12). Much of the current data addresses the effectiveness of early treatment rather than the safety but as yet there has not been any increase in birth defects reported or suggested. Diclectin, in Canada, has particularly been used and studied pre-emptively with no increase in birth defects reported. More research into this developing area is desperately needed.

Finding the Right Treatment for You

It must be highlighted here that treatment for severe NVP and HG should be tailored specifically to each individual patient. There is no 'one size fits all' approach here. Drugs which work for one patient with hyperemesis will not necessarily work for another, and indeed what works for one woman during one pregnancy may not work as effectively in a subsequent one. Sometimes one drug alone won't be effective, but a combination of two or three may work much better.

This is shown quite clearly in a recent survey carried out by Dr Margaret O'Hara through her Pregnancy Sickness SOS site. Of the women who completed the survey, sixty-nine had tried anti-emetic medications with the following results:

- 24 tried only one type
- 23 tried 2 different drugs
- 5 tried 3 different drugs
- 9 tried 4 different drugs
- 4 tried 5 different drugs
- 4 tried 6 different drugs.

These women reported which anti-emetic drugs they had tried and how effective they were, which is shown in the table below. It is important to note, however, that the degree of helpfulness varies greatly, with some women reporting vast improvements in symptoms but others experiencing remaining nausea and/or sickness but to a lesser degree than without the medication.

Name of Drug	No. of women who tried it	No. of women who found it helpful	Success rate (%)
Promethazine (Phenergan, Avomine)	13	6	46%
Cyclizine	46	29	63%
Prochlorperazine (Stemetil, Buccastem)	29	13	45%
Metoclopramide	26	13	50%
Ondansetron	23	20	87%
Ranitidine	7	3	43%
Domperidone	9	3	33%
Steroids	7	4	57%

Even though the drug ondansetron has the best success rate (87%) with cyclizine following with (63%), it should be noted that no single drug is effective 100% of the time and there is no such thing as a 'wonder drug' that works for every woman. Furthermore, there is a hierarchy of drugs which should be followed. Those with the most safety data available and least amount of side effects possible (such as cyclizine) should be used as first-line treatments. Only when these drugs fail to work effectively should other medications (such as ondansetron and steroids) be considered. This is because, although safety data does exist for these, there is much less of it and they carry more problematic side effects for the mother, so it is reasonable to try other drugs first.

Obviously, if first-line drugs are not effective, then it is appropriate to consider trying something else. However, some drugs may have undesirable side effects, which may in and of themselves cause issues (e.g. ondansetron can cause chronic constipation which may aggravate nausea and can be very painful). And in the case of steroids in particular, there is a recommendation that these be retained for the most persistent and severe of cases, and only prescribed after 10 weeks of gestation, when the risk of birth defects drops. Long-term use of steroids has a host of side effects for the mother.

Finding the right anti-emetic for you may be a case of trial and error. As each drug works in a slightly different way, it may be possible to try specific drugs first based on your triggers (e.g. if your major trigger is movement, then an anti-emetic that works well for movement-based nausea may well be a good place to start). This is why it is important to discuss as much as you can with your healthcare provider when trying to decide the best course of action for you.

Alongside the prescription of anti-emetic drugs and antacids, IV hydration should also be considered where dehydration is an issue.

Treatment and Care Plan

Without a clear indication of the cause (or causes) of HG, treatment needs to focus on the management and relief of symptoms. At present, there is no standard approved treatment protocol in the United Kingdom, and with this lack of guidance and no drugs currently licensed for use during pregnancy as treatment for nausea and vomiting, many HCPs are understandably reluctant to prescribe medications unless they deem it absolutely necessary.

This often means the pregnant woman is left to suffer alone until her symptoms become severe enough to warrant hospital admission for IV hydration and even then getting the right combination of medications to adequately manage her symptoms and avoid numerous readmissions can be challenging.

However, this is set to change, and at the time of writing, Green-Top Guidelines are being produced by the Royal College of Obstetrics and Gynecologists (RCOG). These will provide a concise, evidence-based treatment pathway and practical care information for doctors and midwives to treat HG. The authors look forward to the day they can update this book to reflect this development in UK hyperemesis care. In the meantime, we shall continue with the current situation.

Several studies suggest that early intervention may prevent severe NVP leading to the dehydration, electrolyte imbalances, and other complications which are all connected to HG and require hospital admissions. Furthermore, it has been suggested by numerous authors that treatment should be offered to any woman whose symptoms are seriously affecting her quality of life, even if she is not presenting with the more severe clinical signs such as ketosis and electrolyte imbalances.

The United States and Canada both have treatment protocols which are written by professional bodies specifically for the obstetricians and gynaecologists who are likely to treat women with severe NVP and hyperemesis. In the United Kingdom, however, GPs, midwives, and consultants rely on the National Institute for Clinical Excellence (NICE) guidelines to inform them of the best practise when dealing with such cases, and unfortunately, these do not cover the management of HG in such detail.

The NICE guidelines on antenatal care suggest as follows:

'Women, their partners and their families should always be treated with kindness, respect and dignity. The views, beliefs and values of the woman, her partner and her family in relation to her care and that of her baby should be sought and respected at all times.

'Women should have the opportunity to make informed decisions about their care and treatment, in partnership with their healthcare professionals [...] Good communication between healthcare professionals and women is essential. It should be supported by evidence-based, written information tailored to the woman's needs [...] Every opportunity should be taken to

provide the woman and her partner or other relevant family members with the information and support they need.'

The guidelines cover NVP and the potential use of pharmacological treatments for symptoms in section 1.4.1; however, this does not provide adequate detail and information on the safety and importance of treatment in certain cases, nor the need to reassure the patient with HG of this.

'Women should be informed that most cases of nausea and vomiting in pregnancy will resolve spontaneously within 16 to 20 weeks and that nausea and vomiting are not usually associated with a poor pregnancy outcome. If a woman requests or would like to consider treatment, the following interventions appear to be effective in reducing symptoms:

- *non-pharmacological:*
  - *ginger*
  - *P6 (wrist) acupressure*
- *pharmacological:*
  - *antihistamines.*

'Information about all forms of self-help and non-pharmacological treatments should be made available for pregnant women who have nausea and vomiting.'

These guidelines are woefully insufficient to meet the needs of HG sufferers in the United Kingdom. As discussed earlier, the non-pharmacological treatments are well known by sufferers, and there is no attempt by NICE to recognise the severe end of HG. Furthermore these guidelines can actually serve to worsen the HG sufferers' experience as they are often quoted by HCPs when denying women further treatment. The authors are aware of multiple cases in which these NICE guidelines were used to deny treatment beyond antihistamines other than termination.

There is a clear need for easily accessible and recommended guidelines for the treatment of severe NVP and hyperemesis. Sheba Jarvis created a suggested algorithm which was published in the British Medical Journal in 2011 and which is detailed below.

Suggested Diagnosis and Treatment Algorithm (Jarvis)

The healthcare provider should listen to the patient's description of her symptoms, noting that the onset is typically between 6 and 8 weeks of gestation and may include ptyalism (excessive production of saliva), weight loss and muscle wasting, and other symptoms such as abdominal pain, which may suggest an alternative cause.

A full investigation should then be performed when a woman presents with persistent nausea and vomiting which is negatively affecting her quality of life. This should include assessing the patient for clinical signs of dehydration; measuring both lying and standing blood pressure, heart rate, and character; checking the urine for ketones; keeping a chart of the patient's temperature; and weighing the patient weekly. These will help rule out any other causes for the symptoms and ensure that any weight loss, ketosis, or other signs of HG are monitored closely.

Jarvis lists other potential causes for nausea and vomiting as follows:

- Gastrointestinal (e.g. infection, gastritis, cholecystitis, peptic ulceration, hepatitis, appendicitis, and pancreatitis)
- Neurological (e.g. migraine, central nervous system diseases)
- Urinary tract infection
- Ear, nose, and throat disease (e.g. labyrinthitis, Ménières disease, vestibular dysfunction)
- Drugs (such as opoids and iron)
- Metabolic and endocrine disorders (such as hypercalcaemia, Addison's disease, uraemia, and thyrotoxicosis)
- Psychological disorders (such as eating disorders)
- Pregnancy-associated conditions (such as pre-eclampsia and molar pregnancy)

Rehydration should be the first-line treatment, but where nausea and vomiting persists, anti-emetics should be prescribed.

It should be noted that phenothiazine, antihistamines, dopamine agonists, and selective 5-hydroxytryptamine receptor antagonists are all safe in pregnancy and the following anti-emetics are suggested:

- Cyclizine 50 mg orally, intramuscularly, or intravenously, 3 times daily (authors addition – in conjunction with vitamin B6 (pyridoxine) 10 mg orally four times a day)
- Metoclopramide 10 mg orally, intramuscularly, or intravenously, three times daily
- Prochlorperazine 5 mg orally, 12.5 mg intramuscularly or intravenously, three times daily; 25 mg rectally, followed if necessary 6 hours later by an oral dose
- Promethazine 25 mg orally, at night
- Chlorpromazine 10–25 mg orally up to three times daily; 25 mg intramuscularly, three times daily
- Domperidone 10 mg orally, four times daily; 30–60 mg rectally, three times daily
- Ondansetron 4–8 mg orally, intramuscularly, or by slow intravenous infusion, two to three times daily

The healthcare provider should be aware of the potential need to refer the patient to secondary care.

Jarvis notes that if the patient is able to maintain hydration, does not have ketonuria, and is vomiting less than five times per day, then primary care is usually sufficient. This may include prescribing anti-emetics.

However, referral to secondary care (hospital) should be considered in the following cases:

- Continued nausea and vomiting associated with ketonuria or weight loss of more than 5% of the total body weight, despite oral anti-emetics
- Continued nausea and vomiting and inability to keep down oral anti-emetics
- Confirmed or suspected comorbidity (such as confirmed urinary tract infection and inability to tolerate oral antibiotics)

Jarvis expands on this to state that moderate dehydration and urine ketones of +1–2 may be managed with a short admission (4–6) hours in outpatient-based care, whereas severe dehydration with urine ketones of +3–4 (or when outpatient-based care is unavailable), an inpatient admission is warranted.

The algorithm includes further suggestions for inpatient management of HG which includes intravenous infusion of fluids, intravenous thiamine, and intravenous anti-emetic drugs. Whilst in secondary care, a pelvic examination and extensive blood tests (full blood count, urea and electrolytes, liver function tests, calcium, phosphate, thyroid function tests, and serum glucose) may also be carried out.

It is important for healthcare providers to thoroughly assess the patient's symptoms to make the best choice regarding treatment as failure to provide adequate treatment could lead to complications such as

- weight loss (10–20% of body weight)
- dehydration
- electrolyte abnormalities
- hyponatraemia, from persistent vomiting (leading to lethargy, headache, confusion, nausea, vomiting, and seizures), or overzealous correction of hyponatraemia, which can lead to central pontine myelinolysis
- hypokalaemia (skeletal muscle weakness, cardiac arrhythmias)
- vitamin deficiencies (vitamin B1 deficiency can lead to Wernicke's encephalopathy. This may also be precipitated by high concentrations of dextrose)
- vitamin B12 and vitamin B6 deficiencies may also occur, leading to anaemia and peripheral neuropathies
- Mallory-Weiss tears of the oesophagus
- postpartum complications for the mother such as persistence of symptoms and food aversions, postpartum gallbladder dysfunction, and symptoms of post-traumatic stress disorder
- foetal growth restriction and prematurity

There is also research emerging that suggests a higher risk of depression, heart disease, and diabetes in adults whose mother had untreated HG during her pregnancy. However, far more research is needed to investigate the long-term effects, if any, on the infant from poorly managed HG during pregnancy. This is an area the Hyperemesis Education and Research Foundation have been looking into in recent years.

Making It Accessible – A Treatment Ladder to Climb

We have developed the treatment ladder found at the end of this chapter for HCPs to have an easy to follow, visual plan. Start at the bottom and step up each level as required. This can also help sufferers understand the need to start with the lowest required and work their way up.

Conclusion

Since the introduction of IV hydration, HG is no longer the fatal condition it once was. However, this does not negate the need to carefully assess any patient presenting with persistent and problematic nausea and vomiting during pregnancy and treat when necessary with anti-emetic drugs. The trauma caused by such severe symptoms can be immense and complications may be avoided through early and appropriate treatment.

Healthcare providers should be aware of the large spectrum of symptoms and severity of these that pregnant women may experience and be sure to both ask the patient about her symptoms and reassure her if she has any worries. Many women will not mention symptoms of nausea and vomiting as they have been led to believe that it is something they just have to put up with. Reassurance alone that NVP is 'normal' may only strengthen this belief and lead to some patients suffering through severe symptoms, unaware that treatment is available and advised.

When dietary and lifestyle changes alone are not adequate to reduce symptoms, anti-emetics should be offered and reassurance provided that these are considered safe for use during pregnancy, rather than worrying the patient needlessly and making her feel guilty for taking them because of the nature of the difficulty in licensing drugs for use during pregnancy.

Fisk and Atun published a report entitled, 'Market Failure and the Poverty of New Drugs in Maternal Health', which covers this very issue. The lack of research and development of new drugs for any complication during pregnancy has huge implications for maternal care and no drugs have been licensed specifically for the treatment of nausea and vomiting during pregnancy. However, many anti-emetics have been used successfully, without any known risks for decades, and are considered safe for use during pregnancy. These anti-emetics should be offered in the primary care setting, rather than waiting for the symptoms to become so severe that hospital admission is the only option.

It is exciting to note that the last few years has seen a worldwide surge in research into hyperemesis treatments such as using transdermal clonidine in Italy and various other anti-emetics being reported on in research and medical journals. There has been much more interest generally in the subject of HG both in the medical world and in the public media. Therefore, the care and treatment for sufferers can only get better from here.

Finally, the excellent UK charity Pregnancy Sickness Support is working hard to grow a network of peer support volunteers around the country. Contact between the charity, its volunteers, and local GP surgeries and maternity units is a high priority so that women presenting with severe NVP and HG can be put in contact with people who can support them and their families. The information on their website is likely to be more up to date than the information in this book due to the ability to update websites as and when. So it's always worth checking on there for recent research and new treatments.

Following is an example management plan which can be largely filled in by the sufferer and then the various treatments and management strategies discussed and 'signed off' by the doctor. This means the notes can go with the patient and ensure care is provided consistently by doctors and midwives. Alternatively, HCPs can alter it for their specific environment, community, ward, etc. Not all HCPs will be willing to engage in this form of management plan, but sufferers can fill it in and refer to it for self-management. Furthermore, a partner may find it valuable when advocating for sufferers and seeking appropriate treatment. You can download the full document through the Spewing Mummy website to print off or you can photocopy the pages from this book.

A Management Plan for Hyperemesis Gravidarum

To be kept in Patient-held Notes

Estimated Due Date ....

Or LMP ....

This is pregnancy number ....

I have children at home ....

History of twins yes / no

Weight pre-pregnancy: .... KG

Weight now:..KG,

Weight loss to date ....kg (.. %)

Height ....CM

BMI..

I vomit on average ....times per day

I am nauseated .... hours per day

Times my nausea is less bad ....(if applicable)

Current medications I am on, not for hyperemesis:

....

....

....

Adults whom I give permission to discuss my condition with my Healthcare Providers are

....

....

My medical history:

....

....

....

....

....

....

....

....

....

For me the worst symptoms are

....

....

....

....

....

....

....

....

....

....

....

....

Management of Hyperemesis:

First line: ....

Treatment	Tick by patient	Tick by doctor/ script given
Cyclizine (50 mg 3 × a day)		
or Promethazine (Avomine) (25mg 3 × a day)		
And B6/pyridoxine (10mg 3 or 4 × a day)		
Other		

Review of effectiveness, side effects, changes to report:

....

....

....

....

....

Need for antacid addressed and prescribed if required? .... Yes/no

If the condition still worsens, the following criteria will indicate needing to move on:

Symptom	Indication to move on, tick:	Method of monitoring (delete as required):	Agreed by doctor:
Vomiting >5 per day		Patient reporting	
Weight loss >5% of pre-preg weight		Patient reporting/weighing at surgery	
Fluid intake <500 ml per day		Patient reporting	
Urine output <500 ml per day		Patient reporting	
Nausea/vomiting preventing reasonable level of functioning		Patient reporting	
Other			
Other			

If the above deterioration is indicted, I would like to try the following treatments and in the following preferred order (i.e. write first, second, third, etc):

Treatment	Preferred route of administration, delete as appropriate:	Order of preference to try	Tick by doctor and dose/route to prescribe:
Prochlorperazine (Stemetil)	Oral/IM injection		
Metoclopramide (Maxolon)	Oral/IM injection		
Ondansetron (Zofran)	Oral tablets/oral melts/suppositories/ injection		
Domperidone (Motilium)	Oral		
Other ___________			
Other ___________			

Indications for requiring IV Fluids/admission to hospital:

Symptom	Indication to move on, tick:	Method of monitoring (delete as required):	Agreed by doctor:
Vomiting preventing intake of oral medication/not responding to medication		Patient reporting	
Ketones in urine		Patient reporting (Ketostix required)/ urine tested by surgery	
Weight loss >10% of pre-preg weight		Patient reporting/ weighing at surgery	
Fluid intake <500 ml per day, despite medication		Patient reporting	
Urine output <500 ml per day despite medication or not passing urine for more than 12 hours		Patient reporting	
Other___________			
Other___________			

In the event of requiring IV Fluids, in order to avoid admission via A&E, my preferred option is:

Service	Available in area?	Preferred option (write preference first, second, etc)	Doctors comments/ referral to be arranged.
IV hydration at home via local Acute Care Service	Yes/No		
IV hydration as day patient at			
hospital	Yes/No		
Admission to .... hospital	Direct referral to ward available Yes/No		
Other ___________________			
Other___________________			
Other___________________			

In the event of requiring IV Fluids, in order to avoid admission via A&E, my preferred option is:

....

....

In the event of my not responding to treatments so far discussed,

I would like to be admitted to .... hospital to try Steroid Therapy.

My consultant is ....

Telephone/email ....

Self-help I have tried or am using (fill in and tick as appropriate):

Referral to local counselling service to help with the emotional distress caused by HG	Yes/No
I will seek peer support from Pregnancy Sickness Support.	
I will	
I will	
I will	

Treatment Ladder for Hyperemesis Gravidarum

Steroid therapy. Either Prednisolone oral 10mg 3 X per day increasing to 15mg 3 X per day and 20mg 3 X per day until vomiting is controlled OR Hydrocortisone IV 50mg 3 X per day increasing to 75mg 3 X per day and 100mg 3 X per day until vomiting is controlled. Switch to oral prednisolone once oral fluids are tolerated.

Ondansetron 4-8mg oral, IM or by slow IV infusion 2-3 X per day up to 16mg per day †see below for further comment

Domperidone 10mg oral 3 X a day or 30-60mg rectal 3 X a day OR Metoclοprimide 10mg oral, IM or IV 3 X a day (although not suitable for long term use)

Cyclizine 50mg oral, IM or IV, 3 X a day OR Promethazine 25mg oral 4 X a day (Authors addition – in conjucntion with Vitamin B6 (Pyridoxine) 10-20mg oral 4 X a day). *For further alternative options for first line treatments see below.

*Further first-line alternatives include

- Prochlorperazine 5–10 mg 3–4 x a day, oral or 12.5 mg 3 x a day IM or IV or 25 mg rectal once a day.
- Chlorpromazine 10–25 mg 4–6 hourly oral, IM, or IV or 50–100 mg 3–4 x a day rectal.
- Doxylamine 10 mg plus pyridoxine 10 mg up to 8 tablets per day.

† Although many women find ondansetron very effective and recent studies have increased confidence in its safety, the authors come into contact with many women who find the constipation side effect of ondansetron almost as unbearable as the symptoms it is controlling. Bowel management must therefore be addressed when prescribing this, and laxatives should be prescribed where necessary. The severity of constipation should not be underestimated, and it should not be assumed it is due to pregnancy and dehydration when a woman is on ondansetron

Part II

The Hyperemesis Journey

CHAPTER 5

Getting Help: Signs to Watch for and Approaching Your GP

As discussed in earlier chapters, there is no clear distinction for when 'normal' or 'typical' NVP may be progressing into HG. With up to 90% of pregnant women experiencing NVP as one of the most common and expected symptoms of early pregnancy, it can be hard to tell if what you are experiencing is excessive or not.

One of the biggest complaints of women with hyperemesis is that friends, family members, colleagues, and even random strangers can all express that they 'suffered really badly' with 'morning sickness' during their pregnancy. Some of these 'really bad' experiences are then recounted as being sick once or twice a week throughout the first trimester, which compared to a woman who is vomiting multiple times a day, is incredibly mild and even an envious experience!

However, for others 'suffering really badly' may mean that they vomited every single morning for the first 5 months or vomited twice per day throughout the entire pregnancy. And it is important to stress here that, whilst such moderate to severe NVP is not on the same level as HG, there is still a real need to offer support and information to those whose symptoms may not be as severe as HG but still negatively affect a woman's ability to function. Several studies mentioned in chapter 1 have suggested that as soon as NVP begins to negatively affect a woman's life, treatment options should be considered.

But this is where the real difficulty lies: the experience of NVP is so personal and subjective that trying to decide whether your own experience is severe enough to require medical attention can seem impossible. And even if (and when) you decide to approach your GP or midwife, describing the intensity of your symptoms in a way that expresses how severe you find them can be just as challenging. HCPs are aware of the high incidence of NVP in early pregnancy, and without any clear clinical evidence, such as the presence of ketones in your urine, they may well be hesitant to prescribe any medication during those early weeks when the foetus is going through major developments.

So how do you know when what you are experiencing is not 'normal' and you need help?

Well, there are several signs and symptoms that your body may not be coping. The most important sign is perhaps that you feel you are struggling more than you should. Most women expect a certain level of discomfort during early pregnancy, and many have an idea in their mind of what NVP will be like. If you feel that your nausea and vomiting (or either one alone) has surpassed this expectation and is affecting your ability to continue everyday activities such as your ability to eat and drink, leave the house, continue working, or care for older children, then it is always worth making an appointment to see someone.

Studies have shown that early treatment for severe NVP and HG can limit the severity and duration of the symptoms as well as reducing the risk of complications that may arise from associated factors such as dehydration and nutritional imbalances. However, it can be difficult to detect the need for treatment so early on, especially in first pregnancies, due to both the mother and healthcare team attributing the symptoms to normal levels of NVP.

We have already looked at the various treatment options available in chapter 4, so now it is important to look more closely at the signs and symptoms which should alert you to the possibility of HG and the need for contacting your GP or midwife. We will split this into two separate parts: the first looking at evidence that may help you assess the severity of your symptoms, and the second looking at how to approach HCPs.

Signs and Symptoms to Monitor

When you first broach the subject of nausea and vomiting, your GP or midwife will often tell you that these are both 'normal' and 'positive' signs of a healthy pregnancy. It can be difficult to stress just how sick you are, and so it is helpful to know the signs your GP or midwife may be looking for in order to adequately understand the extent of your sickness.

HCPs only see each patient for a short amount of time during an appointment, so they will need to assess the extent of your symptoms rather quickly. Two of the clearest indicators that your sickness is severe are

- weight loss (often of more than 5% of the pre-pregnancy weight)

- presence of ketones in urine samples (this indicates the body is breaking down fat rather than using glucose as a fuel).

Your GP or midwife can check these two things during your appointment; however, you can monitor them yourself at home by keeping a record of any weight loss and checking for the presence of ketones by using a product called 'Ketostix' which are available at most pharmacies and online. (There is a fluid balance chart provided at the end of the book, which you may also find useful for this).

Your GP or midwife will also need to know how your nausea and vomiting is affecting your life, so it is also helpful to make note of the following things:

- When your nausea and vomiting started.
- How many hours each day you are nauseous.
- How many vomiting episodes you have each day.
- How much fluid you are able to drink each day (in a measurable amount such as millilitre, a normal size mug is about 250 ml).
- How much and what kinds of food you are eating each day.
- How often you need to urinate, and how much you produce each time (you can measure this in a cheap plastic jug found in a local cookware store, supermarket or online).
- How much you are vomiting (again, this can be measured in a plastic jug).

These are all measurable indicators of the severity of your symptoms and will offer a much clearer idea of whether medication might be needed than simply saying, 'I have been really sick'. Again, there are charts printed at the back of the book which you can use to monitor these.

Finally, it is important to mention to your GP or midwife how your symptoms are affecting your ability to function. How would you answer the following questions?

- Are your symptoms affecting your ability to function normally?
- Are you symptoms affecting your ability to do paid work?
- Are your symptoms affecting your ability to care for your family?

- Are your symptoms affecting your ability to care for yourself (e.g. wash yourself, prepare your own food?)
- Are your symptoms affecting your mood (are you feeling anxious, de pressed, isolated?)

Make a note of your answers and take them with you whenever you see your GP or midwife and note whether these change from day to day and week to week.

The Pregnancy Unique Quantification of Emesis (PUQE) Score

The Motherisk Program in Canada has produced a unique way of assessing the severity of sickness using a specific series of questions that focus on the length and frequency of certain symptoms. This easy-to-use system may be useful for you to use in conjunction with your doctor or midwife to monitor your sickness regularly.

In the table below, mark the answer to each question which best describes your own experience, and then use the scores next to each of your answers to give you a final 'score'. (Also available in Appendix 2 for you to photocopy).

Pregnancy Unique Quantification of Emesis and Vomiting Score (PUQE) – over 24 Hours	
In the last 24 hours, for how long have you felt nauseated of sick to your stomach?	Please circle the one answer
Not at all	1
1 hour or less	2
2–3 hours	3
4–6 hours	4
More than 6 hours	5
In the last 24 hours, have you vomited or thrown up?	Please circle the one answer
I did not throw up	1
1 to 2	2
3 to 4	3
5 to 6	4
7 or more times	5
In the last 24 hours, how many times have you had retching or dry heaves without bringing anything up?	Please circle the one answer
No times	1
1 to 2	2
3 to 4	3
5 to 6	4
7 or more times	5
On a scale of 1–6, how would you rate your nausea and/or vomiting today, if 1 is acceptable and 6 is extremely debilitating?	Please circle the one answer 1 2 3 4 5

The idea behind this system is that by combining clearly quantifiable symptoms (such as vomiting and retching) with more subjective symptoms (experience of nausea), you get a better picture of the overall effect the symptoms are having on your day-to-day life. In particular, the combination of subjective and objective (or quantifiable) symptoms may help your healthcare provider to determine the best course of action to take. So, for example, a woman who is vomiting less frequently but suffering highly in terms of how the nausea is affecting her life may need different treatment to one who is vomiting multiple times each day but is not so distressed by the nausea.

What do you do if your GP or midwife refuses to acknowledge the severity of your sickness or offer treatment?

As always, it is important to reaffirm here that if you feel that your sickness is excessive and affecting your quality of life, then you have every right to ask for a second (or third or fourth) opinion. Nobody knows how much your symptoms are affecting you better than you do, and you should trust your own instincts on this. Obviously, it is important to discuss everything with your GP and/or midwife as they are there to offer support and guidance; however, it is unfortunately not uncommon to come across a healthcare provider who is unaware of the impact of and treatment options for severe NVP and HG.

If you are unhappy with the outcome of any appointment you make, remember that you can ask to see a different GP or request a referral to a consultant who may have more experience in this field. It might also be useful to take someone else with you to any appointments so that they can advocate for you. Sometimes it can be incredibly difficult to express everything you need to when you are feeling so rough. There is guidance for partners to advocate on your behalf in chapter 7.

The charity PSS has a list of 'HG-Friendly' GPs and consultants and may also be able to provide you with someone in your area who might be able to help. Outside the United Kingdom, the HER Foundation can help source doctors experienced in treating HG effectively. Contact details for both charities are provided at the end of the book.

Approaching Healthcare Professionals

> *In my first pregnancy, I had no help or acknowledgement from any healthcare professionals. It wasn't until I was in hospital after the birth that I was diagnosed with hyperemesis. They thought I was on [recreational] drugs, and I had to argue that I was so thin because of how much I'd been vomiting. In this pregnancy, the healthcare professionals have been amazing and understanding. They even helped me with some of the remaining issues I had from my previous HG pregnancy.*

(Debra, HG Sufferer)

Talking to HCPs about pregnancy sickness and hyperemesis can be difficult, though it varies a lot. There is currently a lot of misunderstanding about hyperemesis, and archaic misconceptions about psychological causes and physical or mental weakness are still held by many otherwise excellent doctors, nurses, and midwives. The Thalidomide disaster in the 1960s was truly awful, and fears about medicating in pregnancy, which stem from that, are still widely held, particularly about medicating for pregnancy sickness. Interestingly, there are plenty of other pregnancy conditions which are happily medicated without a second thought as well as numerous non-pregnancy-related conditions, experienced in pregnancy, for which medication is standard. For example, steroids for asthma or Crohn's disease are standard. If you needed an appendectomy and happened to be pregnant, you would likely be pumped full of anti-emetics and pain relief without mention of need verses risk.

But it is important to understand where HCPs are coming from too. Doctors, nurses, and midwives are registered professionals who take personal responsibility for their actions, omission, and prescriptions. Most live in daily fear of being sued or struck off their professional register and are overworked and underpaid considering their responsibilities. On top of that, GPs are under pressure regarding prescription costs and admission figures. Often this balance is not well thought through due to lack of time, and if they medicated early, HG symptoms could be more effectively managed meaning they could reduce the admission figures and ensuing cost. But it's just not that easy to weigh up in the middle of a busy surgery, and if they don't come across hyperemesis very often, it can be hard to appreciate the impact.

> *My GP in my third pregnancy was amazing. She was so kind and sympathetic. Plus she was thorough with her care and treatment. We made a plan together before I got pregnant, and it made such a difference. The pregnancy was still awful but at least I wasn't battling to get treatment too.*

(Amy, HG Survivor)

A lot of how well your GP responds will depend on how you approach them. If talking is difficult for you, try to have your partner or another friend or relative with you. There is advice about how they can advocate for you in the section for partners. Here are some ideas about how to approach your GP:

- Go in with a good attitude. Don't assume that the doctor will be dismissive, and don't assume that you will have to 'fight' for treatment. If you are reasonable, then they will have a hard time explaining why they are being unreasonable.

- Start with explaining why you are there, perhaps try: *'I do not think that what I am experiencing is just morning sickness. My symptoms are much more severe. I have been unable to keep down food and water, and I vomit continuously throughout the day. I am concerned for my well-being because I'm getting dehydrated and losing a lot of weight.'*
- Prepare yourself in advance with some information about HG, perhaps print some information from the PSS website. Take notes in with you, in particular about your symptoms, your concerns, and any questions. Specifically, how many times were you sick yesterday, how much fluid you kept down. What self-help have you tried, and did it help. For example *'I've tried eating little tiny bits often as advised, but it just comes back up. I've been resting, but I'm sick even when lying still'.*

This table can help you prepare for an appointment in advance:

Symptoms:	How many times a day are you vomiting? How much fluid and food have you kept down in 24/hours? How often are you passing urine? Have you lost much weight? What other symptoms are you experiencing, for example, dizziness, headaches, etc? Is movement, sound, and smell triggering vomiting?
Your concerns:	What are your main worries? That you are severely dehydrated? That you have lost so much weight? That you are bed-bound and getting sores or at risk of DVT? That your baby is at risk from the dehydration and starvation? That you are getting depressed from the isolation and relentless sickness? That you are going to lose your job over this?
Questions:	Is it safer to take medication or not? If you are not being admitted now, then at what point should you be concerned that you need to go to hospital? What signs and symptoms should you look out for that things are more serious? What is the best route for speaking to the GP? Can you email or phone to speak to them? Could you monitor your ketones at home? Are there other medication options and routes, such as, injections, suppository, melts?

If you can, take a urine sample with you so it can be checked for ketones and the concentration can be checked.

Make it clear that you understand the medications aren't licensed for pregnancy but feel that when looked at from a risk/benefit perspective, you think the time has come to accept that you need treatment. Explain that you had hoped to have a nice natural pregnancy, without medication, but that your symptoms are so severe you think the risks of not treating outweigh your desire for a natural pregnancy.

Try also to be sympathetic to their prescribing budgets. Point out that a hospital admission would be far more costly and that you are willing to arrange collection of repeat prescriptions on a regular basis so they can just do shorter prescriptions, for example, a week or 10 days' worth at a time. That way if you change medications, get miraculously better, or sadly miscarry, then you won't be left with hundreds of pounds worth of medication in your cupboard. A willingness to compromise is always appreciated.

Now assuming your doctor has reacted really well and is being kind and proactive, ask for a plan going forward. He doesn't need to agree to more medication or anything else just yet, but he needs to let you know what symptom severity to look out for and when to come back if things don't improve. If he is sending you home rather than to hospital, then ask what he would like you to monitor, for example, fluid intake/output, weight loss, ketones in your urine – he can prescribe Ketostix for this, or you can buy them yourself online.

Recognise too that getting the treatment right can be a case of trial and error, so always ask for advice on how long to give the medication to work and what to do if there is no improvement, or you get side effects or your symptoms get worse. GPs can feel frustrated if a patient is expecting a cure from them when there is no cure to give. Accepting that there is no cure, yet, and that you need to look to 'manage' the condition will help a lot.

The aim of the game is to build up a team feeling with the GP and make it clear you want to work with them to manage your condition and you don't expect a quick solution from them.

> *My experiences with healthcare professionals were generally good. Although to start, the GP wouldn't prescribe medication, she was incredibly sympathetic and shared her own stories of how sick she felt when pregnant. She also said I could come back just to talk to her and moan about*

how I was feeling. She said if it progressed and got worse, she would review the situation regarding medication.

(Hazel, HG Survivor)

Hopefully, by following these steps, you will develop a good working relationship with your GP and feel that you have received good treatment and support. But what if it doesn't go to plan as above? What if despite your careful description of symptoms and your concerns, you are still met with 'It's normal' or 'No medication is safe in pregnancy', 'You're just pregnant', and so on?

Well, if the doctor is trying to claim it is normal, then ask at what point they would consider severe nausea and vomiting to not be normal and what level of dehydration they consider acceptable for a pregnant woman.

If they give you a lecture about taking medication in pregnancy and claim it isn't safe and that you might be damaging the baby, then ask for the evidence base for such claims. Point out that there is far more evidence that not treating HG effectively has greater risks for the baby and mother than treating with medications for which there is no evidence of adverse foetal outcomes (you might want to write that down).

If they are just nervous treating pregnant women, then ask for an urgent referral to a consultant or suggest they phone a local consultant for advice.

Remember that GPs generally don't know what the next patient to walk through the door is suffering with until they sit down and tell them. Hyperemesis is not particularly common with many GPs seeing one or two cases a year, and they can't keep up to date with all of the research about every condition. So try to be sympathetic to that, perhaps signpost them to the PSS website where there is a section specifically for HCPs to read about treatments and perhaps offer to give them some time to look into the options. You could phone back in the afternoon or pick a prescription up later (making an effort now to be flexible will pay off in the long-term).

Ultimately though, if you don't feel you've been treated well or received the help you need, then ask to see someone else. Go out to reception and ask for another appointment with someone else. If you have the strength and feel you have grounds, you could ask to speak to the practice manager or make a complaint. But keep it in perspective. Getting treatment needs to come first and complaints are often more stressful than they are worth. Remember also you are entitled to change GP practice.

You can also get in touch with PSS (or the HER Foundation outside of the United Kingdom) who know of 'HG Friendly' doctors and HCPs in your area they may be able to put you in touch with.

Other HCPs can be just as problematic, and you are likely to come in contact with nurses, midwives, hospital doctors of all levels, consultants, and possibly dieticians and psychiatrists. But remember plenty of HCPs are wonderful and caring, and as awareness and understanding about hyperemesis increases, so will the standard of care and treatment.

> *The midwives in hospital were often patronising and treated me like a small child, telling me my husband had 'done this to me' and it was 'all his fault'. That kind of 'naughty him' humour is not very funny when you haven't eaten for two weeks.*

(Lina, HG Survivor)

> *At week 18, I saw a dietician. 'I hear you've been a little sick and aren't eating enough,' was her opening gambit. Had I not been attached to a drip and feeling so weak I would have liked to smack her! On the other hand, the midwives were all fantastic. I was in and out of hospital the whole of my pregnancy so I got to know them all. And my consultant was amazing. He got me through the pregnancy undoubtedly. Although he admitted it had been a while since he had seen a case as bad he did get me through to 37 weeks.'*

(Katrina, HG Survivor)

Even if your symptoms do not seem as severe as someone else's, or you are worried that everyone else is right and you are just making a fuss over nothing, please do consider going to visit either your GP or midwife.

CHAPTER 6

Coping Strategies[*]

Resigning myself to doing nothing and putting my life on hold for the whole pregnancy. Staying in bed every day! Buying ready meals for my family to eat – employing a cleaner! Asking my husband to make ice pops so I could get a little liquid down. Not feel guilty about just eating what I could even if it wasn't healthy food. They are the ways I coped.

(Leeanna, HG Survivor)

This section contains information that may help you to manage your symptoms and hopefully get on with life as best you can. You haven't got hyperemesis because of anything you have or haven't done, so none of these strategies will cure you. They may, however, help you cope better both physically and mentally with the symptoms.

Remembering that pregnancy sickness affects women of all personalities, ethnic backgrounds, and types of environment is helpful in reducing the isolation and the feeling of fault or blame that some women feel. It can be hard not to feel isolated and guilty when you are told that 'If you'd only think positively, you'd be okay! Get out for some fresh air.'

Pregnancy sickness on any level can be very unpleasant indeed, but when it becomes so severe, it is classed as hyperemesis. It's far more than just unpleasant. It's bordering on torture! However, even at the point when NVP affects the quality of life of the woman, treatment should be considered.

It felt like I had drunk poison, like my insides were rotting. I was dizzy when I stood up and my husband would have to help me on the stairs. The movement would trigger vomiting though. I could vomit continuously for 30 minutes or more. It was torture!–

(Amy, HG Sufferer)

If you are suffering from, or think you are suffering from HG, it is important to contact a GP as soon as possible. In the event of an emergency, contacting your GP and/or going to a hospital emergency department is important. As discussed already, dehydration and starvation can be serious and help should be sought.

I was worried about asking for help. I thought I was being a wimp. Loads of women get morning sickness and they just cope. I couldn't understand how they had coped, but a lot of my friends were telling me that they had still managed to go to work. I thought what I had was worse but I had never heard of anyone suffering so bad before so I thought it was just me... being weak.–

(Laura, Severe NVP Sufferer)

If you have 'normal' pregnancy sickness, you'll be pleased to know that it usually settles by 12–14 weeks of gestation – but then you probably aren't reading this book if you are suffering from 'normal' pregnancy sickness. Hyperemesis, on the other hand, tends to continue to around 20 weeks, although for a lot of women with hyperemesis, symptoms will still remain at full-term. Some women have the full severity of symptoms throughout the whole pregnancy, but this is not as common, and generally, there is an improvement from around 20 weeks. Either way, 20 weeks is a long time and it's worth having some strategies up your sleeve.

Coping with other people

The lack of understanding is probably the most stressful aspect. Obviously, the vomiting and exhaustion is horrendous but to have people treat you like you're making it up or somehow faking it for attention is crushing. Especially when you genuinely feel like you may not survive the pregnancy.

(Debra, HG Sufferer)

Women who suffer hyperemesis often find it difficult to communicate the severity of their condition to others, particularly to those who have never heard of it and may have preconceived ideas about 'morning sickness'. You may find it helpful to have a speech prepared for when people ask you about why you are ill. If someone asks what is wrong, give them the benefit of the doubt that they haven't heard of hyperemesis and are genuinely interested in your well-being. PSS suggests you could try responding to them as follows:

'I have a medical condition called hyperemesis gravidarum. A lot of people think it is like morning sickness, but in reality, it is much more severe. Although most pregnant women feel nauseous during their pregnancy,

most pregnant women do not have this condition – it's a rare complication.'

Talking to family and close friends about hyperemesis can be difficult. Your partner and other loved ones may feel like there is nothing that they can do to help you and that in itself can be stressful and upsetting for them. Let loved ones know that their support means a lot to you and you appreciate it. Suggest that they read the section in this book written for them in chapters 7 & 8. You can also print off the information for family and friends from the Spewing Mummy and PSS websites.

Suffering from NVP or HG can be a lonely and emotional experience. People may say things to you that clearly demonstrate they do not understand what you are going through. Here is a list of the sort of things you may well hear during your pregnancy with hyperemesis and the replies you can keep up your sleeve for when you need it:

'*Have you tried ginger ?*'... This has got to be the most commonly reported thing women hear. As discussed early in the book, ginger may well help with mild nausea, but if you're throwing up night and day for weeks on end, then it really is unlikely to help and could exacerbate symptoms with painful reflux. Response suggestion by Lina – HG Survivor: *'Ginger only works for mild nausea in concentrations of 1,000 mg. It's not regulated, and anyway, would you want to puke stuff that burns when it comes up?'*

'Oh I had that, but I still went to work and got on with life.' Remember that pregnancy sickness is on a spectrum and has a whole range of severities from a mild whiff of nausea around week 8 to life-threatening vomiting for 9 months. Your friend is likely lucky enough to have never suffered any illness to this degree and therefore can't understand the variation and severity. A good line in this situation is 'Well, that's like comparing a twisted ankle to a broken leg'.

'Think positively and get some fresh air.' The implication is that it is all in your mind and you are causing your own suffering. It's a terribly cruel thing to say and can cut deep, especially if said by a well-meaning loved one. Generally, though, this comment is truly meant well and is often said by people who really want to help but don't know how or what else to suggest. A response would be along the lines of, 'If thinking positively helped, I wouldn't have this awful illness, I was really excited to get pregnant.'

'*Well, at least you can get pregnant, you should be grateful for that.'* This can really add to the guilt some women already feel. Many women experience negative feelings towards the pregnancy, and a perception of 'not being grateful enough' can exacerbate that significantly. Plenty of women with HG have even been through the pain of both infertility and hyperemesis and are pregnant thanks to IVF. So the hurt for them is all the more.

This comment is hard to respond to, particularly if it's from a friend who is struggling to get pregnant or going through IVF, because she genuinely would swap places with you in an instant. How you respond to this will differ quite a lot depending on who said it in the first place. If it is someone who has genuinely experienced the heartache of infertility or pregnancy loss (or who desperately wants a child and is unable to for any other reason), then you might try saying something like, 'I am sorry that you feel I am not grateful to be pregnant, because I truly am. I know how much you would love to be in my position, and I sincerely hope you get the opportunity one day to experience a healthy pregnancy. However, I am so sick and I am scared about how sick I am and so that makes it hard to express my gratitude for being pregnant.' You may also like to add something along the lines of, 'I don't want this to come between us, so can we talk about how we can support each other through this?'

However, if the comment comes from someone who has a family of their own and they are just being particularly heartless, you can afford to be a little bit more forthright with your answer and might like to try something along the lines of, 'I know how lucky I am to be pregnant and I am extremely grateful, even if it doesn't appear that way to you. Would you like to ring me and tell me how grateful you are you had kids next time they bring home a sickness bug and you just want to hug the toilet?'

'*I loved every moment of pregnancy. It's such a special time, creating life, glowing blah blah blah blah.'* The authors recommend avoiding this friend or relative until your baby is here at which point they'll probably be really helpful with nappy changing and rocking. But if ignoring them isn't an option, then perhaps try explaining, 'I'm really pleased for you. That is how I imagined pregnancy would be for me too but it has been torturous, scary and depressing. I would appreciate if you could be sensitive to that'.

'*Is it safe to be taking those drugs? Won't they harm the baby?'* Remember, no woman actually wants to take medication in pregnancy. We all (well most) go into pregnancy wanting to be natural earth mothers, eating healthy and avoiding all potential harm, but sadly some women cannot survive pregnancy without medication. In the past, before the invention of modern medicine, women would simply die often without knowing why as symptoms would kill her before a pregnancy was confirmed or even suspected.

Many women with HG who are taking medication think dozens of times everyday about the safety of what they are taking. They question if they really need them and if the baby will be okay. The reality is the drugs are prescribed by a doctor and given because they are needed. They are ultimately safer than not taking them. Perhaps question back, 'If I was having an asthma attack, would you question if the inhaler was safe? No, you'd be pumping away worried that I may die without it!' Point concerned relatives in the direction of PSS, the HER Foundation, or hand them this book.

> *I remember at 39 weeks having a complete panic about whether the baby would be okay. Not because I was worried about the medication I had taken, I knew it was safe from the research I'd read, but because if there was anything wrong with the baby, I knew people would say it was because I had taken medication. They wouldn't remember that I had needed the medication to maintain the pregnancy and avoid dying. They would just see the defects regardless of the cause.*

(Amy, HG Survivor)

When people make these comments, try to remind yourself, 'They mean well, but they do not understand. I did not understand before I had this experience'.

> *People used to say I should stop thinking about it and I wouldn't be sick, that it was mind over matter. In the end, I just stopped talking to people, which became more isolating. But it was easier than having to deal with other people's views. I'm normally a very strong person, but being that unwell, I didn't have the energy to cope with them.–*

(Mandy, HG Survivor)

Joining online forums can help you connect with other women who are going through or have been through a similar experience. Sharing 'war stories' and awful comments can really help. Both PSS and the HER Foundation have forums you can access.

Coping Out and About and Staying In

Many women who are suffering from NVP or HG become afraid of leaving their homes, worrying that they will be unable to control their vomiting in public. As a result, they may feel socially isolated, unable to spend time with their families, friends, or co-workers who they used to see on a daily basis. It is important to try to continue to interact socially. If you do not want to leave your home, it may be helpful to try to call a close friend or family member with whom you can talk or text. Using other forms of social media, such as Facebook, Skype, or FaceTime, can also help you to remain connected with your outside world.

> *My first pregnancy was before the invention of Facebook or smart phones. I had to use a computer to log onto a forum. Well, that was impossible anyway! By the time I got pregnant again, I had a smart phone and had connected with hundreds of women on Facebook and the Pregnancy Sickness Support forum. It really helped with passing the day. I could use my phone in bed lying really still just using one finger, and I felt much less isolated.–*

(Amy, HG Survivor)

Being in touch with a PSS volunteer can really help with the social isolation being housebound can entail. We talk more about the volunteer network later and contact details for them are in the appendix.

Accepting that you are going to need help during this phase of your life may help you to come to terms with your experience. It can be difficult to ask for help with tasks you never had trouble with before; however, accepting that you need help may increase your ability to cope better and reduce the severity if you can just rest as much as possible.

If you are able to get out of the house, or if you have to go for doctor's appointments, scans, and so on, then you may find it helpful to carry a 'sick kit'—a small pack of wipes or tissues, some sick bags (disposable nappy bags are good), a small bottle of water, and some mints or lemon sweets.

Some women find it easier in the car if they are driving, while others prefer to be a passenger (especially if you are likely to vomit).

It is a good idea to empty your bladder before going out and regularly whilst out. Relaxin, the hormone produced in pregnancy, can cause havoc with bladder control during episodes of vomiting! Incontinence pads can also offer significant security if you are worried about weeing whilst vomiting not just out and about but at home in bed too.

Being bedbound and reducing the risk of DVT

Women with the more severe end of the NVP spectrum and HG may find they are literally bed-bound for weeks on end and with that comes increased risk of complications such as Deep Vein Thrombosis (DVT) and pressure damage. A DVT is a blood clot which can form in your legs or pelvis and if it breaks off from the vein and travels to your lungs it can cause a potentially life-threatening condition called Pulmonary Embolism (PE). Pregnant women are already at increased risk of DVT due to various physiological changes in your body during pregnancy, such as increase blood volume, and women with HG are at even more risk due to dehydration. So it is important you try to reduce the risk as best you can. If you are admitted to hospital you may be given an injection daily to combat the risk and you may be provided with special knee or thigh high stockings to wear. You can take these home and continue to use them if you want and if you are too ill to do the following risk-reducing steps then it is a good idea to keep them on.

- Switch between bed and a chair on a regular basis
- Getting up and walking around your bed or house as often as possible
- Do simple leg exercises such as flexing and extending your foot, rotating your foot in circles.
- Stretch your thigh muscles (hamstrings) while lying in bed – raise one leg in the air as high as you can (up to a 90 degree angle), pull the leg towards your body gently and hold for 30 seconds. Release gently and repeat with the other.
- From a lying position bring one knee to your chest, hold for 15 seconds and release slowly, repeat with the other.

Ultimately for the women with severe hyperemesis all of those above prevention measures may seem impossible and you should discuss your risk with your GP or midwife if that is the case. They may prescribe compression stockings at home for you. But knowing the signs and symptoms of DVT and PE is very important for bed-bound pregnant women and should you experience any of the following symptoms then get rapid medical assessment:

- Pain like a heavy ache, swelling or tenderness in one of your legs (usually your calf). The pain may be worse when standing or walking.
- Red or noticeably warm areas on your leg, particularly at the back of your leg below your knee
- Swelling in one area or on one leg

For symptoms of DVT see a doctor as quickly as possible.

Sometimes a DVT won't have any symptoms and you could suffer a PE with no prior warning. The symptoms to be aware of for PE are:

- Breathlessness, either coming on suddenly or gradually
- Chest pain, which may be worse when you inhale (breath in)
- Sudden collapse

For any of the symptoms of a PE you need to call for an ambulance.

To reduce the risk of pressure damage try to change position regularly (every two hours or more frequently) and try to make sure there aren't creases in the sheets where you are lying. If you are very concerned or are developing pressure sores, which start as red patches that don't go white (blanch) when you press on them, then speak to your doctor or practice nurse.

Coping with Excess Saliva

It is a little discussed problem and one which many women don't realise is actually common. Suffering in silence thinking they are some sort of salivating freak of pregnancy serves only to add to the misery. But it is very common for women with hyperemesis and also very distressing. It's so common and 'real' that it actually has a name: Ptyalism.

The distress from this symptom is complex. On the one hand, the psychological impact of knowing you are already very dehydrated and yet losing even more precious fluid through excessive saliva production is frustrating and confusing. And then, of course, is the embarrassment caused by the bizarre condition and resulting dribble, not to mention the sometimes necessary 'spit cup' which is carted around with you to the doctor's surgery, by your hospital bed, or to the sofa on the rare occasion a friend visits (putting them off returning any time soon).

But what if you don't spit it out... ergh, swallowing it is even harder when you have hyperemesis! Many women report that attempts to swallow the excess saliva results in more vomiting.

What can you do about ptyalism? Well, sadly, there is no actual cure or remedy. So, like most symptoms of hyperemesis, it's a matter of management. There is a little anecdotal evidence that omeprazole, which you may be prescribed for acid reflux, may help a little with this symptom also. Although this is yet unproven as the medication is already used in holistic HG management. However, as studies have so far found no adverse effect on the foetus, it may be worth discussing with your doctor.

Simply knowing you are not alone with this symptom will, hopefully, help with the psychological aspect. As you read this, there are literally thousands of pregnant women in the United Kingdom and indeed all around the world spitting into cups or towels or futilely repeating the cycle of swallow and vomit. Perhaps try connecting with a few of them via such groups as the PSS or HER Foundation forums. If there isn't already a thread for excessive salivation, then start one and share horror stories and coping tips. Honestly, it helps to know you are not alone.

A lot of women suggest using an opaque cup with a lid to spit into and find that effective. Others use a towel and switch it when soaked. Others use a combination of tissues and cups. When you can eat, then dry foods might help dry your mouth temporarily and bring some respite. Rinsing your mouth regularly might help and will at least alter the taste. Different flavours will work for different people, but things like lemon water or soda water may be worth a try too. Unfortunately, like most aspects of HG, you'll likely find what helps you personally through trial and error.

Whatever you do, don't avoid fluids in the hope of reducing the saliva. It is a sure fire way to end up on a drip, or worse, and it won't work anyway.

A little good news about excess saliva is that it may help to protect your teeth from the damaging effects of the acidic vomit and help prevent decay. It's not much compensation, but it is a little.

Coping Mentally

NVP and HG can be very traumatic. The physical and mental stress on the sufferer and her partner can be profound. Vomiting and prolonged retching can result in a suffocation sensation that can feel like torture and be deeply traumatic. Relationships can become strained under the pressure the situation puts on both partners. Women can feel a complete loss of control, as their lives turn upside down and are unable to care for themselves or anyone else for months on end.

Traumatic symptoms, such as flashbacks, intrusive images, nightmares, numbness, depression, and a tendency to feel withdrawn, are not uncommon experiences during or after hyperemesis due to the extreme nature of the symptoms. These symptoms can continue for some time after the baby is born, and research by the HER Foundation in America has found an increased risk of post-traumatic stress symptoms after a pregnancy complicated by hyperemesis.

Research suggests that the following may help with trauma:

- Give yourself permission to look after yourself.
- Try to process your experience through an artistic outlet such as writing about it or painting an image of your experience. Try to write in the first person and present tense and use as much detail as possible.

If traumatic symptoms persist, it is very important you seek professional help. There is more information in chapter 11 and links to further help in Appendix 1.

Strategies to cope mentally vary from person to person, so some of these suggestions may work for you or they might not be 'your thing'. There is no harm in trying different strategies though.

Talking to others about your condition can be very challenging. Many people do not understand the severity of hyperemesis. As mentioned above, having a speech prepared to answer questions about your condition can be helpful, as can reminding yourself that they are not trying to be unfeeling – they may just not understand. Talking to people who do understand can be wonderfully supportive and really help to reduce the mental isolation and suffering. Luckily, in the days of easy internet access, you can get support via online forums, Facebook, and Twitter. A list of social media contacts and forums is in Appendix 1.

You can also reduce the isolation by getting in touch with the charity PSS which has developed a fully insured network of trained volunteers to offer one-to-one peer support to sufferers. Support is usually via text or email, but you can also speak to a volunteer on the phone, or if you live close by, you may be able to arrange a home visit. All of the volunteers have been through hyperemesis and have had further training via the charity, so they can appreciate the trauma specific to hyperemesis. If you are outside of the United Kingdom, then get in touch with the HER Foundation for help and support.

> *My husband was amazing, and contacting Pregnancy Sickness Support was the best thing I could have done. It was hard to look at a screen for very long, so emailing, texting, and even talking on the phone was hard, but just knowing there was someone there who cared, understood, and would text/email weekly (even when I didn't respond) made me realise I wasn't alone.–*

(Mandy, HG Survivor)

You may find it helpful to keep track of how you are feeling throughout the experience, both physically and emotionally. Keeping a diary or journal of your experience may be helpful for several reasons. This will also allow you to look back and see how far you have come.

> *In my first pregnancy, I got a sort of blank pregnancy calendar from a pregnancy magazine. I used to cross off the day before I went to sleep each night and I'd write in when I had milestones like scans and when I felt the baby move. It was great getting to the end of a month and turning the page. By the third trimester, although I was still very sick, I could look back and remind myself of how far I had come and how much better I was than in those first few months. That really helped me–*

(Amy, HG Survivor)

You can get a Spewing Mummy Calendar from the website accompanying this book on which you can cross off each day as you get through it. It won't actually help your symptoms, but it may help psychologically to track your progress through the 9 months.

A diary can help you to process your experience, enabling you to make sense of how you are feeling and of what this experience means to you as a part of your life. Many people who suffer from medical conditions find that reflecting on their experience, through writing about it, helps them to make some sense of such an experience. An online blog is easy to set up and can be kept anonymous or completely private although many sufferers would find typing or writing just too much while they are seriously ill.

> *During my second pregnancy, I had a huge notice board up on my bedroom wall where I could see it. I had pinned pictures of where my husband and I want to have our second honeymoon (the first had been ruined by HG), baby scan pictures, and a list of all the things I was looking forward to eating and drinking again! Every morning when I woke up faced with yet another day of hyperemesis, I could focus on all the good things to look forward to once the baby arrived and it was enough to make me get out of bed every day! And when I finally got the things on the list, it was like being in heaven!*

(Katie, HG Survivor)

Try to envision the end point and remember that this is a part of your life and remind yourself as often as necessary that

- this condition is not your fault.
- you have not done anything to cause hyperemesis.
- there is nothing you could have done to prevent the onset of hyperemesis.

It can be easy to feel sad that you are not having the ideal pregnancy you had hoped for. Women are sold lots of ideas in our modern society, and having a perfect happy pregnancy is one of them. Disappointment over the loss of a good pregnancy is natural. However, everyone has a different story, and your story involves hyperemesis. It's also natural to feel jealous of other people's pregnancies and even resentment towards your partner for not being the sick one. Give yourself a break and accept that it's okay to feel these things, but try to remember it's not their fault either.

I felt such resentment towards the baby. People would ask me all the time if I was excited and would go on about how I would fall in love with it straight away. They would tell me about how they thought it was magical feeling a baby move inside them. I always thought I would too... but I didn't. I just hated it. I wanted it out. I fantasised about miscarrying and terminating. I'm ashamed to admit it now. I love my son so much. But there is so much pressure on women to enjoy pregnancy. It's nonsense. When you feel sick constantly, getting your stomach kicked from the inside by your baby is like torture – I felt like my baby was torturing me.

> *In my last pregnancy, we knew what to expect and it was a whole different experience. I saw hyperemesis as a monster and it was trying to take my baby – I had to fight it. I saw that it wasn't the baby's fault and it wasn't the baby making me sick; it was the HG. That really helped me, and I never once thought about miscarrying or terminating. I saw myself as a HG warrior, and I was fighting for my baby. I wasn't going to let the HG win.*

(Amy, HG Survivor)

Feeling resentment to your unborn baby is not something that many women like to talk about. It's taboo. But the reality is that a lot of women with hyperemesis do feel negative feelings towards the baby. It's understandable as if you weren't pregnant you wouldn't be sick. The negative feelings towards the baby in turn lead to guilt for having those thoughts in the first place, and it can all compound already depressive moods. But as the quote above says, if you can try to see the HG as a separate thing to the baby, it may help you cope and reduce those negative feeling.

> *I thought about terminating in the early weeks. My husband was going on a business trip, when I was 11 weeks. So I booked into a clinic, with the idea of telling him I'd miscarried. The night before he went away, I broke down... I didn't really want to go through with it, but I didn't know what else to do. It was a crazy idea really, how exactly did I expect to be able to get to the clinic... I could barely lift my head off the pillow, let alone get in a car!*

(Anon, HG Survivor)

> *I would say the hardest part of it all was that I hated my baby. My sister had given birth to her little girl a year earlier, and she had told me that she wrote letters to her baby when she was pregnant. Every night I would try to write a letter to my baby and I couldn't think of one thing to write that was nice. Not only did I hate everyone for not believing me, for not understanding me, but I hated my baby. I didn't think I would be able to love her because of how sick she had made me. I hated all of it. But the day she was born was the best day of my life, and the first time she looked at me, I*

knew that it was all for something so special and that I would never hate my baby again.–

(Ashley, HG Survivor)

Distracting yourself from the situation is likely to help with not just passing the time but reducing the time you can spend nurturing negative feelings towards the baby, your friends, partner, HCP, yourself, and your situation. It may not help with the nausea and vomiting symptoms, but it is likely to help with the mental impact of the isolation and depressive moods.

What you can do to distract yourself will depend largely on your personal symptoms. In the early days, you may only be able to lie still in a darkened room. TV and reading may be out of the question but could a gentle audiobook on a quiet volume pass the time while you lie there?

As the weeks go by, you may find you are able to read, use the internet, and watch TV. You might find an e-book reader, such as a Kindle, easier to tolerate as it is lighter than a book and doesn't require page-turning. You can also access new books instantly from your bed and switch between books, magazines, and newspapers without getting up. Avoid depressing books about miserable situations! Try comedies and light-hearted literature as they are more likely to improve your mood rather than darken it. Factual books about things that interest you or quirky and strange short stories may be a good distraction.

Smart phones have revolutionised the experience of being bed-bound, and you can access forums and friends from bed using one finger to navigate the screen.

I found solitaire on my phone would pass hours and if I got really nauseated after some food in the last trimester, I would lie on my side and play it. It took enough mental concentration to distract me from the nausea and pass the time, but it only required me to move one finger, and it wasn't overstimulating with bright colours and flashing lights.–

(Amy, HG Survivor)

Coping with Eating and Drinking

I had to be amused at the two pieces of paper given to me on admission to hospital for hyperemesis. The first one was advice about HG which stated that six small meals a day are far better than three larger ones. The second said, 'Meals in this ward are served at 8 a.m., 12.30 p.m., and 6 p.m.'!

(Hazel, HG Survivor)

Many women find there is a time each day when their symptoms are less severe, so keeping a daily diary of your symptoms may enable you to be prepared to eat and, most importantly, drink at those nausea-free times. Some people have found that the diary helps them to become more aware of their nausea-free times. The worse the NVP, the shorter these nausea-free intervals are, so it is important to be as ready as possible for them. Sometimes you may even feel hungry, but the hunger is often quickly followed by the onset of nausea. So, either feeling hunger or a nausea-free interval gives you a chance to eat straight away. Knowing when these times are can help you to make the most of these opportunities. If you cannot face a meal, keep nibbling your favourite food, especially when nausea threatens. Women with moderate NVP say that eating, especially small frequent meals, and stopping eating as soon as your stomach feels full is the most successful way to improve their symptoms.

In my first trimester, when my symptoms were at their absolute worst, I found I had around a 15–20-minute window in which I felt well as soon as I woke up. It was just enough time to get out of bed, stumble downstairs, make some instant porridge or heat up some rice pudding in the microwave, and start eating. The nausea would build up incredibly quickly and would already be threatening by the time I made it downstairs and into the kitchen. But I knew it was my only chance in the day to try and eat something, so I would work as quickly as I could and then eat as much as I could before the nausea became too great. Most of the time, I would only manage half a bowl of porridge or half a pot of rice pudding before I had to give in, but I always saw that as an achievement. If all I had was 15–20 minutes each day, then I was not going to waste them!

(Amanda Shortman, Author and HG Survivor)

Unfortunately though, many cases of hyperemesis don't allow for any eating at all as literally everything comes back up. This can be particularly difficult to manage. If you are able to try tiny bits, then do as it will help prevent some of the more serious complications and will make it easier to keep on top of things as you get better. It's also still worth trying to keep a diary of symptoms to help you monitor your condition to find out if there is even a small window of opportunity to try to consume some foods and liquids.

Despite the intense and constant nausea, every so often I'd get sharp pains of hunger as well. I found that particularly distressing because if I ate to calm the hunger pangs, I'd vomit almost immediately and both the nausea and hunger would still be there. But then my throat would hurt too and I would go back to just lying as still as possible.

(Amy, HG Sufferer)

Keeping a fluid balance chart is really helpful too and may aid in discussions with healthcare providers. There is a chart you can copy from this book or download it from the Spewing Mummy website.

Eat whatever you fancy (within current guidelines for pregnancy). Hopefully, you have a super supportive and helpful partner willing to dash to the shops at 9.30 p.m. to get you gherkins, salted crisps and frosties, or some other odd combination. Because weirdly women with hyperemesis can still suffer cravings and that in itself can be really horrendous when mixed with constant nausea.

More common with hyperemesis though are food aversions, and these can be tricky to manage particularly when they strike in the middle of eating the food which you suddenly become averse to! What appeals one day can absolutely revolt you the next.

At first certain food and drinks were craved – such as Orange Fanta! She was getting through four to five cans a day just to take away the metallic taste. Trying to be practical, I looked around all the supermarkets and found one that had an offer on Orange Fanta. I purchased thirty cans to get us through a week and save myself from nipping to the corner shop at 21.55 p.m. Well, did this backfire or what! This craving was very short-lived, and after having Orange Fanta coming out through her nose the taste and smell was the worst she had ever had and couldn't stomach another can or even look at one – so there I was stumped with twenty-eight cans of Orange Fanta. This was not my only "bulk-buying" disaster. They ranged from having seventeen bags of Walkers Chunky Ridge Salt and Vinegar through to various chocolate bars and biscuits.

(Matthew, HG Partner)

You'll likely soon discover the foods which stay down better and the ones which come back up less unpleasantly.

> *I used to judge food on how bad it would be to vomit it up. Tea and toast isn't too bad, but cornflakes were awful and pasta kind of dries out, so I felt like I was choking as I'd bring it back up. That was what food had become to me... vomit.*

(Amy, HG Sufferer)

> *I made a game out of seeing how good things tasted on the way back up. Sounds ridiculous, but it was a case of if I didn't laugh, then I would never stop crying!*

(Debra, HG Survivor)

Fortifying food: Although you can buy pre-mixed fortified drinks such as Ensure or 'build up' type products designed for people with compromised nutrition they are not all suitable for pregnancy. Some of them contain levels of vitamin A over the recommended dose for pregnant women. You can however fortify milk yourself by adding 4 tablespoons of milk powder to 1 pint of full cream milk. This milk can then be used for drinks that you find tolerable such as milkshakes, hot chocolate or smoothies, or use it on cereal or in puddings, porridge or jellies.

If you are managing to eat small amounts at your family mealtimes then try to add calories to your meal by fortifying with hard or pasteurised cheese, butter, crème fraiche, margarine, meat and so on.

Tips for fluids: Many women find lemonade or fruit drinks easier. Sucking ice cubes or nearly freezing fluids can help. You can buy ice lolly moulds that you make at home with squash or just water. Some women find the smell of tap water really strong in pregnancy, so a filter or buying bottled water in bulk may help. Some women find drinking through a straw or from a sports bottle helpful.

Alternating between eating and drinking may help you keep food and fluid down, rather than having a drink at the same time as food. Space them out.

Rehydration salts can be a really good way of gaining maximum benefit from what little fluids you can manage. They contain electrolytes which are lost through excessive vomiting. Because of the level of glucose in the mixture, the osmolarity of the liquid is identical to plasma and this in turn increases the absorption of sodium and water. You can buy sachets to make up a mixture, and you need to make sure you make it up to the correct amount of water.

You can also make your own by mixing 1 litre water with 6 teaspoons of sugar and ½ teaspoon of salt. The quantities are important as if it's too strong, it can actually reduce the absorption of water. Better to err towards a weak solution if in doubt.

Personally I (Caitlin) found rehydration salts more palatable than plain water, but unfortunately, for some, the flavours of the bought ones can be triggers for vomiting. You could try making ice lollies out of the mixture though or using your own recipe and adding a sugar-free cordial for flavour (if you add a cordial that contains sugar, you'll alter the quantities in the recipe above).

To estimate how much you are drinking, measure how much liquid your favourite cup/mug holds and then judge from that. For example, if your husband fills your mug that holds 200 ml and you've drunk half of it, then you know you've had about 100 ml. Bottles of mineral water can be useful for that too. You can judge if you've kept down a whole 500 ml bottle, only half of it (250 ml), only a quarter (125 ml), and so on. It can be encouraging to see how much you've managed to keep down. But it can equally be a warning if you don't manage a certain amount in a day.

Coping with Odours

Smells can be a big problem for the hyperemesis sufferer! There are a few things you can try though. The smell of cooking, especially fatty foods, coffee, tea, cigarette smoke, or perfume are the most common triggers. You might also find that the smell of your husband turns your stomach or even the smell of your other children, which can be particularly distressing.

> *In my first pregnancy, my husband had to change deodorant three times and eventually got an odour-free one. Sometimes he had to sleep in the spare room partly because of the movement on the bed but mainly the smell. He doesn't smell bad normally, and I was so upset trying to explain to him. I wasn't rejecting him and it wasn't his fault; I just couldn't help it.*
>
> *In my next pregnancy, he would bring our son in to see me for 10 min-*

utes when he got home from nursery, and a couple of times, I started retching from the smell of my 18-month-old son, so my husband would take him away again. It broke my heart. I found it was worse if he had been given food with garlic in so we spoke to the nursery and they agreed to make sure garlic wasn't in any of the food until I was a bit better. Also his clothes would smell odd. I think it was from the perfume from a staff member at the nursery, so daddy would get him changed as soon as he got home. It all sounds so drastic now, but it was terribly upsetting at the time.

(Amy, HG Survivor)

Eating cold food can reduce the smells in the house; hopefully, your family will agree to do the same. Normal smells can become unpleasantly nauseating, making shopping and cooking impossible. Lower your standards for a while. If your older children are in school and if they can have a cooked school meal, then they could just have sandwiches in the evening. Accept any offers for your children to eat at friends' houses, especially if they'll drop them back afterwards. Weekends can be a good opportunity for your partner and children to go to a friends for Sunday dinner and leave you at home to rest. You may feel sad and lonely that you aren't there with them, but once this is over, there will be plenty more opportunities. If friends ask how to help, suggest having your partner and kids over or ask them to make a meal for your freezer.

It's not unheard of for the partners of hyperemesis sufferers to be found microwaving their dinner outside the back door or in the garage!

You could also try to find things which help mask unpleasant odours with smells you can cope with. For example, a little lemon, lavender, rose, or peppermint oil on a tissue, or whatever smell you personally can tolerate could help.

You can also buy unscented soaps, deodorants, and washing powders which may be helpful.

It can be particularly upsetting if the smell of your partner or a previous child is triggering retching and vomiting, but please know you are not alone and this is not uncommon. Reassuring your partner that this happens for a lot of women and encouraging them to read the partner's section of this book may reassure them that it's not actually that they smell, rather that your nose is the problem. It may be particularly bad in the first trimester, and you may even find they need to sleep in a different room. This particular symptom does tend to improve though, so reassure them that they won't be banished for long. It will help if they don't smoke, eat garlic, use strong deodorants, and so on.

Oral Hygiene

Brushing your teeth while you have HG can become your most dreaded time. It is a very common trigger for vomiting, and many women report it as an ongoing trigger after pregnancy if the toothpaste foams too much or a particular brand of toothpaste is used, etc. Oral hygiene can rapidly become a source of great worry and added stress for sufferers. Women report not being able to brush their teeth at all for weeks or months, and there is the obvious damage that can be caused by acid erosion on the enamel of the teeth with prolonged and regular vomiting.

So what can you do to look after your teeth as best you can during the hyperemesis pregnancy?

First of all, it's important that you do not brush your teeth immediately after vomiting. This may seem counter-intuitive, and you may desperately want to freshen your mouth up at that point, but brushing can further erode the enamel already weakened by the acid in the vomit. Instead, rinse with plenty of water to wash the acid away.

You can get fluoride mouthwashes that may help as well. Those aimed at children are likely to be more tolerable and possibly more effective for remineralising the tooth enamel. If you can tolerate chewing gum, then get one with Xylitol in. Xylitol actually helps to stop plaque adhering to your teeth, so if you can't brush your teeth, then this is the next best thing.

Also, if it is the toothpaste foaming up that is the main trigger, then don't use toothpaste, or get a low-foaming one (many of the organic and natural ones don't foam very much). Electric toothbrushes tend to cause far less foaming than manual ones. They are more effective at cleaning your teeth, and they take much less effort on your part – no arm jiggling! That said, the vibration may end up adding to the nausea or triggering vomiting.

If the only drinks you can manage are sugary, then try using a straw as this will reduce the harm these drinks cause to your teeth. Many women find using a straw easier anyway.

Ultimately, it's a matter of doing what you can, when you can, and not beating yourself up if you can hardly do any of the above. Make sure you get a thorough check-up and deal with any problems as soon as your pregnancy is over, and take advantage of the free NHS treatment you get for a year after pregnancy.

Vitamins

You are meant to take a pre-pregnancy prepared multivitamin that contains 400 mg of folic acid daily, during pregnancy. Some research suggests that iron tablets can make NVP and HG worse, and some women find it easier to avoid vitamin tablets with iron included. However, some women need iron tablets for specific conditions such as anaemia, which can be common in pregnancy.

Folic acid is most important in the very early days, and the recommendation is only until 12 weeks although most women (ones without hyperemesis) take them throughout pregnancy these days. Folic acid has been found to significantly reduce the risk of neural tube defects such as spina bifida and other serious conditions. The neural tube forms very early in pregnancy, days 26–28, which is before you generally know you are pregnant, so supplementation during the trying-to-conceive phase is the really important time. Folate (vitamin B9) is an essential nutrient found in green, leafy vegetables, broccoli, peas, corn, oranges, grains, cereals, and meats, so if you had a healthy balanced diet before finding out you were pregnant, then the risks of you being deficient are far lower.

Pregnancy vitamins can be a source of huge guilt to women with hyperemesis, who find them completely intolerable. Try to keep them in perspective. We all go into pregnancy thinking we'll take them every day, and we won't take medications or try a sip of alcohol or stand near a smoker... but we're not all able to take them and some of us need medication, so give yourself a break – at least you won't be having any wine or seeing any smokers while you're house-bound!

Rest

Rest helps, preferably lying down or propped up with pillows, probably on your side. Pregnancy sickness is like motion sickness in many ways, so even small movements of the head, as in brushing your teeth, can make it worse. Lying down doesn't work for everyone though, and certainly, lying down flat can exacerbate reflux. In that case, try to find positions that you can keep still in and which are comfortable, perhaps on the sofa or a comfortable chair. There are also all sorts of weird and wonderful pregnancy cushions on the market that may help you get comfy.

If rest works for you, then try to arrange your day so that you get as much rest as possible. Sadly though, resting as much as necessary while you are suffering badly can make women feel guilty. If you do feel guilty, try to remember that rest is important for you and your baby. It is your pregnancy, and you need to look after yourself. It's not uncommon to hear things like 'You're just pregnant and pregnancy isn't an illness.' Well, it's true, pregnancy is not an illness, but HG is an illness, and it's a serious one.

> *Staying in bed and trying to sleep as much as possible was the only thing I could do. I realised quickly that I couldn't keep up my personal hygiene standards.–*

(Lina, HG Survivor)

Coping with Employment

> *I fell pregnant just 5 weeks before my wedding, and HG kicked in 2 days into our honeymoon. When we arrived home and I was immediately signed off sick for a week, my employer thought that I was 'faking it' to get an extra week off. I had told them I was pregnant before leaving, but it made no difference. They even called to say that they had done some investigation and seen that my husband was off as well one day that week (he had a bug so had taken a sick day). I then endured very nasty comments on Facebook from colleagues about having a 'long honeymoon' and eventually I asked my GP to write a letter to my employer explaining what I had. The sucking up and apologising I got later that day was enough to win an award. After that they couldn't do enough to help!*

(Katie, HG Survivor)

Five separate medical studies have shown that 30% of pregnant women in paid employment need time off work due to NVP. You are not alone if you require sickness benefit because of NVP! Employers also need to recognise that about 8.6 million hours of paid employment are lost each year in England and Wales due to pregnancy sickness. Several medical studies have shown that in excess of 50% of women with severe NVP struggle with their usual daily routine as housewives and mothers. Accept whatever help is offered. Indeed, organise the help if you can! If you have hyperemesis, remind yourself that this is a serious and debilitating condition, and it is your right to take time off work and you have the right to not face discrimination or unfavourable treatment.

In the United Kingdom, at the time of writing, the Equality Act 2010 states that it is unlawful discrimination for an employer to treat a woman unfavourably because of her pregnancy or an illness relating to her pregnancy or because she is exercising, has exercised, is seeking, or has sought to exercise her right to maternity leave. This special protection applies from when a woman becomes pregnant and continues until the end of her maternity leave, or until she returns to work if that is earlier. This is referred to as 'the protected period'.

Anyone who has suffered discrimination can bring a claim for compensation before an employment tribunal.

Discrimination could be demotion, dismissal, or the denial of training or promotion opportunities because an employee is pregnant or on maternity leave. An employer can't take into account any pregnancy-related absences during the protected period for the purposes of attendance management or when deciding whether to dismiss an employee as it would be considered unfavourable treatment. Therefore, any sick leave taken for a pregnancy-related illness should be recorded separately by your employer.

> *I'm a nurse and was told that every pregnant woman gets sick and I should just get on with it. My director of nursing wanted me to be disciplined for my sickness record!*

(Amy, HG Survivor)

Unfavourable treatment for any of the following reasons will amount to pregnancy discrimination, although this isn't exhaustive:

- any absence due to pregnancy-related illness
- a woman's inability to attend a disciplinary hearing due to pregnancy sickness or other pregnancy-related conditions
- performance issues due to pregnancy sickness or other pregnancy-related conditions

The employer has to know, believe, or suspect the woman is pregnant for their unfavourable treatment to be unlawful. Whether they know by formal notification or through the grapevine, once they know you are pregnant, you are protected by these laws. You don't actually have to tell them you are pregnant until 15 weeks before your due date (25 weeks pregnant), but it's in your interest to notify them as soon as possible so the legal protection is triggered.

For more information about your rights to maternity leave, sick pay, and if you are facing unfair dismissal or pregnancy-related discrimination, please see the links in Appendix 1.

You may also need to look into childcare options. What options you have will depend very much on where you live, and it's a good idea to ask around family and friends for recommendations and advice. Your partner could help with arranging childcare, and reminding him/her that if you get admitted to hospital, they will have to take time off to sort out the other children may be a good incentive for them to take the reins. There is further information about the childcare options in the section for partners. Under new laws in 2014, no one can be discriminated against because of someone else's pregnancy and this could be very relevant if your partner is having problems with their employer.

Remember though, not all employers are difficult or unsupportive.

My employer was very supportive. My working hours were reduced immediately on return to work and I was checked on regularly to make sure I was okay. I can't fault my employer.–

(Kat, HG Survivor)

I was so lucky with my employer. They were very supportive and never made me feel guilty about being off sick. They were very helpful with making sure I got the statutory sick pay I was entitled to, and they were as flexible as possible with my hours for the few weeks I was well enough to work. I never got any snide comments from colleagues either, they were all very sympathetic. -

(Amy, HG Survivor)

Conclusion

How women cope with the trials of hyperemesis and the various symptoms, both physical and mental, that it entails is very individual. What works for one woman may not work for another.

Finding your own coping strategies is important though, and asking your partner, family, and friends to support your coping strategies is important too.

Making contact with other sufferers is likely to really help as is the old adage of eating little and often when possible and resting as much as you can.

Try to remember that you will get through this and you will be a stronger person for it.

> *Hyperemesis is a truly bonding experience. At the time, you may feel totally alone and isolated and find it impossible to believe that anyone else has ever suffered like you are doing, but they have, and are, and will. Connecting with other sufferers is an incredible experience in itself and to find out you are not the only one who has fantasised about miscarrying a baby you tried for months to conceive and you're not the only one being told to think positively and try ginger, is liberating. By bonding with other women, you can gain hope and a strength to survive the condition. United we can make a massive difference not just to our own experience but to thousands of other women too. I now have friends not just around the UK but around the world, women and their partners whom I am bonded to by hyperemesis gravidarum.*
>
> *Through hyperemesis, I have learned compassion and tolerance and gained an inner strength which I honestly didn't have before. Hyperemesis sufferers may feel totally alone and misunderstood by healthcare professionals and the world, but we are not alone. There are literally hundreds of misunderstood conditions which are met with equal disbelief, pseudoscience, and old wives' tales. For example, myalgic encephalomyelitis, fibromyalgia, various allergies, irritable bowel syndrome, symphysis pubis dysfunction to name but a few. At least with hyperemesis, it's generally over in 9 months. Many other conditions last a lifetime! Hyperemesis has given me an insight into suffering without compassion from others and made me a better person for it.*
>
> *I lost a few friends over my experience but not many and far fewer than many women I know who simply couldn't cope with how abandoned they felt by their friends. I did feel abandoned too by many of my 'close' friends and relatives. But then I gained perspective and came to realise that it's simply impossible to understand if you haven't been through it and it's not*

through lack of caring... It's a lack of knowing how to care. When you are the ill one, stuck in bed day after day, week after week, it's hard to remember how quickly the weeks fly by when you're at work every day, sorting the kids out and generally getting on with life – it's a matter of perspective. See tolerance and perspective as things you will gain from this experience and you'll be grateful for it in the long run.

By the time I gave birth, I was weak, physically and mentally. I had barely moved for 9 months let alone exercised. After nine long months, I was at breaking point, and every day was as much of a struggle to get through as in the first few weeks. But once that baby comes out I'm ready to take on the world. Maybe not physically, I can barely walk up the stairs without getting out of breath, but mentally. Bring it on! Nothing seems as hard again. I know it's not as easy for everyone, and the mental health legacy from hyperemesis can be profound, but luckily for me, the strength it gave me has been brilliant – Think of it like a hardcore workout at the gym. It's not much fun while you're there, but you come out a lot stronger.

(Caitlin – HG Survivor, Author)

CHAPTER 7

The Partner's Experience

It is common for hyperemesis to be seen as a problem only for the woman suffering, but the partners of sufferers will know only too well this is not the case.

In reality, partners and their experiences vary widely. In our experience, we have come across women with the most incredible supportive partners and women whose partners have up and left at the very first vomit, unable to cope. It is our hope that the 'partners' reading this section, be they husbands/boyfriends, wives/girlfriends, mothers, sisters, or best friends, will be of the supportive variety and that by reading this section, they will feel less alone and more empowered in the knowledge they are doing all they can for their loved one.

> *It is horrific to watch and emotionally draining. I hate seeing her so vulnerable and helpless as it really is not in her nature or character. I do help as much as I possibly can, but it can be extremely frustrating and feels as though there is nothing more I can do on the days when she is having particularly bad episodes.*

(Fadhili, HG Partner)

It can be hard for the partners to admit that they are struggling with the condition because they know only too well it is easier for them than the sufferer. That said, many partners genuinely wish they could switch with their loved one and take the suffering for them. Often this is compounded by the feeling that their partner, the sufferer, would be doing a better job of looking after them and the house and any other kids. Of course, that's not always true, but we hope in this chapter to try to verbalise some of the emotional roller coaster partners can go through during the long months as a carer.

It is not uncommon for relatives, friends, and complete strangers to make ignorant comments about how it's actually harder on the partner, and of course, the sufferer and her partner know that's not true. However, it is extremely hard on the partner of a sufferer and there can be no denying that!

In first pregnancies, it can be a scary thing to witness your partner deteriorate, become dangerously dehydrated, and bed-bound. It is commonly reported by partners that they would rush home in lunch breaks to check on the sufferer with genuine fear of her dying.

In second and subsequent pregnancies, if there are already children to be cared for, it can be a whole new world to a dad who, in effect, becomes a single parent and carer quite suddenly. Learning to juggle getting the kids to nursery or school, sorting out the washing and cooking, and shopping on top of having to go to work to pay the mortgage really is no easy feat. Partners must be careful not to burnout and get depressed. You can quickly become exhausted if you are doing everything without help or without your own support system.

> *The hardest aspect is the fact that I work a full-time job and feel like there is hardly any rest for me. I get home from work after long hard days and it's straight to cleaning up, emptying sick bowls, putting on laundry loads, preparing dinner, putting our 6-year-old in the bath and getting her ready for bed, and only then does the thought of finally just sitting down and zoning out cross my mind.–*

(Fadhili, HG Partner)

Feelings of guilt and helplessness are common in the partners of women with HG. It is half their baby after all and perhaps they had wanted the baby more than the suffering woman initially. But tackling the pregnancy as a team and supporting treatment plans, decisions, and situations will ease this.

In this section, we hope to suggest ways that as a woman's partner, you can support her and survive the situation. Some of the things will not be relevant to your situation, and some may sound so obvious it's bordering on offensive. It is not meant that way, but sadly, not all partners are helpful and supportive and some need things spelling out. If a suggestion seems offensively obvious, then give yourself a pat on the back and feel reassured that you are already a really great partner.

A partner not supporting his/her wife can be hugely detrimental as resentment is quick to build, and trust can be rapidly and irreparably broken when a partner is unsupportive, questioning the illness or treatment and unhelpful with practicalities. Paradoxically, by reading this chapter, you are already demonstrating that you want to help and support and that you believe in her suffering. And in those relationships, hyperemesis can have a long-term bonding effect giving your partnership a strength beyond that imaginable pre-hyperemesis.

How to Support Your Partner

It's as much about what not to do as what to do when it comes to the patient with hyperemesis. Emotions are as frayed as they are ever likely to be. She is emotional not just because of the hyperemesis: the normal pregnancy hormones cause mood swings and emotional instability all on their own. Trying to take things in your stride and not rise to provocation is key! Deep breaths and understanding that it is not her fault but rather the powerful hormones combined with the torturous situation will help you get through each day. And that should be your goal – getting through each day, one day at a time. On the bad days, just take it an hour at a time.

> *Chin up, get on with it, be their rock, and don't take any enforcement of physical distance personally. If you need help, ask for it.–*

(Soren, HG Partner)

So let's start with a few basics of what to do and what not to do. Some of these will be very obvious to the majority of readers of this book, and it's a shame that they don't go without saying. But they don't!

First – Not Being Phased!

Throwing up can be embarrassing. Even more embarrassing is when, at around 20 weeks pregnant, you start to wet yourself whenever you vomit. Your partner is likely to experience this and is likely to feel really embarrassed the first time it happens. If you handle it right, hopefully, she will be able to laugh about it in the future. If you want to be a really great partner, you'll help her clean up and then you'll pop to the shop, discreetly buy some size small incontinence pads, and subtly leave them in her underwear draw.

Sometimes the vomit may miss the target and splatter the walls, floor, bedspreads, and her pyjamas. It might stink too... it's grim, but if you can just clean it up without letting on that you're grossed out, she will appreciate that, and again, you may both be able to laugh about it afterwards.

Emptying sick bowls isn't much fun either but being sick in a bowl is often preferable to the toilet, so not seeming phased by this chore is a good move. Keeping the toilet spotlessly clean is also a must.

> *One time, she was vomiting so hard she peed on the floor and on my foot. She got up and went to lie down. I just took my sock off and got on with cleaning the puke-covered toilet. Then, when she got her strength back, we had a good laugh about it. That's how you get by. You don't make a fuss. You just smile and know that when you look back on this, you're going to laugh about it a lot. I mean, how could you not?–*

(Chris, HG Partner)

A quick note on toilet cleaner at this point. If it is possible to get a fragrance-free cleaner, then that might be your best bet; otherwise, you may find you have to change products regularly as the smell of the toilet can rapidly become a trigger. The chemical smells, like bleach, can be really heightened during pregnancy, so natural ones may be gentler on the sensitive nose. Other women will like the smell of bleach, as it can instil confidence in the cleanliness of the toilet bowl. Bear in mind though that if using bleach, be careful to flush it away thoroughly as a vomit episode causing splash back could be a disaster – bleach in her eye really is the very last thing she needs right now!

Managing Dehydration and Treatments

Signs of dehydration or severe illness to watch for include the following:

- Persistent vomiting four or five times per day
- Dry mouth and lips
- Passing only small amounts of dark urine, for example 500 ml or less per day
- The loss of 5%, or more, of her pre-pregnancy weight
- The presence of ketones in her urine.

If you want to monitor her fluid input/output or ketones yourself, then you need to buy a cheap measuring jug and some Ketostix. (You can buy them at a chemist or order online, see the Spewing Mummy website for links.)

To measure fluid balance, she will need to wee in the jug every time so you can measure it (note also the colour. If it's very dark, then she is dehydrated), and you will need to provide drinks in a measurable way, for example, a 500-ml water bottle, then estimate how much she has drunk, say half (250 ml) or quarter (125 ml). A household mug is about 250 ml. (If she has a particular cup or mug, you could measure how much it holds to be sure). Document everything in and out for 24 hours and then add up the totals. If her input or output is less than 1,000 ml, you need to think about treatment, but if it is less than 500 ml, you should consider trying to get her admitted to hospital for IV fluids. There is a fluid balance chart in Appendix 2, or you can download it from the website.

To measure ketones, your partner will again need to wee in the jug or another clean vessel. Take the lid off the Ketostix, take one out, and then shut the lid again. Don't leave the lid off the sticks because it can compromise their accuracy. Dip the test end in the urine just for a second so it is wet and then wait for the result for 15 seconds. To read it, you compare the colour to the ones on the pot. If your partner has ketones in her urine, you should speak to her doctor because she may need admitting for fluids.

Medications can be tricky to manage, and some women end up on a whole variety of drugs. Different medications work in different ways, so treatment plans which combine therapies tend to be most effective. Unfortunately though both the hyperemesis and some of the medications to treat it will make her drowsy and potentially confused. This can make remembering her medications tricky. A tip is to get a dosing box from the chemist which has compartments for morning, noon, afternoon, and night for the 7 days of the week. Once a week, you can fill the little compartments with the various medications she is on and set reminders on her phone for while you are out at work. That way if she can't remember if she has taken her last dose, she can just check in the pot and she doesn't need to remember what to take and when. There is also a drug chart in Appendix 2 and on the website you might find helpful to use.

Helping Around the House

Rest is an absolute must for the hyperemesis sufferer. You may notice a correlation between days where she feels a little better and so does a few extra things, tries to tidy up or go for a short walk, and a rapid deterioration either that evening or the next day. This is really common and demonstrates the need for her to rest even in her better moments. She mustn't feel under pressure to help out around the house just because the nausea has waned for 2 hours or the new medication is helping a bit. She is likely to put plenty of pressure on herself anyway. You may be desperate for her to help out as she may do household tasks a little better or more efficiently than you feel you do and you're most likely feeling swamped by it all. But try to resist asking her for things.

> *I feel that even after everything I do around the house in order to keep things running as smoothly as possible (which some might say should just be done and not moaned about), I am taken for granted. A thank you would make a world of difference. Even 'How was your day today?' I do understand that as men, we will never fully understand the extent to which our partners are suffering with this condition. But we are here for them. It's frustrating that even after all we do, even just a thank you is sometimes forgotten.*

(Anon, HG Partner)

There are a number of things that can help you manage the household chores, but it may depend on what you can afford. Shopping can be ordered online and delivered at evenings or weekends when you are home to unpack. The fridge may be a no-go zone for her, so this would be really helpful. If you can afford a cleaner, then that could be a good option for some families. There are laundry services too in most cities and larger towns. They will pick up dirty washing and drop it back a couple of days later clean and ironed.

If you have children already, then lowering your standard of family meals for a few months won't actually harm them in the long run. Ready meals in the freezer are great, and fish fingers, chips, and beans a few nights in a row isn't that bad in the greater scheme of things and is very quick for you to organise after you've been at work all day. If your child goes to nursery, then you may be able to arrange for them to have dinner there which will make things a lot easier. Take up any offers from family and friends who want to give you a lasagne or casserole or who are happy to have the kids (and you) round for tea. People are often keen to help but don't know how and providing food is a great way for them to help you out. If they ask how they can help, then suggest a meal for the freezer (Remind them to go easy on the garlic though!).

Smells

Smells are a major problem for the patient with hyperemesis. Her nose is like that of a bloodhound, except it's not just hypersensitive: once pleasant smells can suddenly become revolting. Supporting her in avoiding the need to go near the fridge and cutting out coffee at home may be easy enough and obviously cutting out cigarettes and garlic are basic requirements. But what about when the very smell of you, or of your child, turns her stomach? That can be deeply upsetting.

She will be just as upset by this as you are and you must try not to take it personally or get defensive. It may be little things that are easy to change such as finding an odour-free soap to wash with and a perfume-free deodorant. Even a little garlic in your diet can make you smell awful to the hyperemesis sufferer and you may need to ask the nursery to avoid this in the children's food or otherwise go to the effort of making packed lunches for the children.

Too much beer is also likely to make you smell bad, and as mentioned above, cigarettes are a big no-no (but then you'll be giving up for the baby anyway right?).

> *I have gone through seven different deodorants during this pregnancy, and at present, I'm currently using Nivea Silk and Smooth 48 hour (yes, it's a women's one, but I can confirm it smells nice and works). At one point, my deodorants were located on top of the fridge as I had to spray them outside. I have since moved to roll on and now women's deodorant. Back in the day, Channel Platinum Aftershave would send my fiancée into a frenzy and make her drag me upstairs and make me late for work, but now it sends me to the naughty step for being stupid by spraying it in the house. I now have a stock of deodorants in the car (2 of which I can't use!) and 2 aftershaves.*

(Matthew, HG Partner)

Ultimately though, you could make all sorts of lifestyle changes, change your soap, deodorant, shaving gel, laundry detergent, and so on and the smell of you could still be too much. Particularly at night and early morning when body smells are concentrated. If this is the case and she would prefer you sleep in the spare room or sofa, try to understand it is only for a short while and not meant personally. She will appreciate your help and understanding. This is an aspect many partners really struggle with as they feel so rejected, so we hope by reading here that it is normal you will feel reassured that it's not you... it's the HG.

Food smells are a big problem, and you may need to accept that cold meals are the way forward for a short while. Cold meats, cheese, bread, and salad may be your staples for a while, and in the summer, that's easy enough. In winter, you could try soups which don't tend to smell too much if you just heat them enough to be warm. Some partners have resorted to running a lead outside to microwave their tea in the garden or garage. It sounds a bit drastic, but if it avoids an evening of constant vomiting, it's probably worth the effort.

Sex and Intimacy

Now, most of you will know that at the end of the day, sex is not the be all and end all and that if your partner is sick, the last thing she wants to do is have sex! Unfortunately, there are a number of people out there who require it so frequently that even if their partner is sick, the pressure is on to perform. A woman I supported once said despite her husband being otherwise very supportive, helping with the children and housework and so on, she was still having to have sex a few times a week despite being so sick. Her husband 'didn't mind if she needed to stop to be sick... a bowl was by the bed'. Masturbation wasn't an option because her husband believed 'in a marriage that's like cheating'. Well, let us spell it out right now: it is not cheating! It's absolutely fine, and if it means your sick wife doesn't have to make herself sicker, then just get on with it. Pressuring your partner into sex when she is ill is far more disrespectful in a marriage, than attending to your own needs.

Intimacy, on the other hand, is something she may well be craving. The long lonely hours in bed and the feelings of distance from the entire world can be overwhelming, and lying together (if she can cope with the smell) holding hands and talking can significantly improve her mood and reduce her loneliness. As with all aspects of support though, it needs to be dictated by what she can cope with and wants.

Providing company for your partner will ultimately foster intimacy between you. Remember to text her from work to remind her that you love her. She probably won't be feeling very lovable at the moment, and a lack of intimacy is likely to compound that. Reminding her that you love her regardless and that together you will get through this will mean so much more to her during the long lonely hours at home than a quick 'I love you' as you both departed for work did in the days before HG. It may be a different sort of intimacy compared to the fun times of trying for a baby, but there will be plenty of time for that in the future, particularly if the relationship is nurtured now and the nightmare of hyperemesis is used to foster a strong team spirit and mutual respect for each other's suffering and strengths.

A note on sex and intimacy after HG

Many couples experience a lull in their sex life while they have very small babies, which is understandable given the sleepless nights and step up in the general pace of life as new parents. In addition, women can have issues around body image and lack of confidence with their post-pregnancy bodies and there may be issues with scarring around her vagina or labia from the birth which can cause discomfort during sex. Sensitivity to these particular issues is necessary in all relationships, but the partners of women who experience HG may be faced with a more specific challenge to their love life... a fear, or even phobia of pregnancy.

And it is not just the women who may experience anxiety around the act which ultimately causes HG for her, men can too and it is totally understandable! This topic is discussed in more depth in chapter 10 so if either you or your partner are struggling with this particular aspect of recovering from HG then please turn to that chapter and have a read of how to help.

> *We didn't have sex for ages again as I was so worried about getting pregnant again despite having a coil. I've now had the coil out and my sex drive has gone up but my partner is terrified I could get pregnant again and won't come near me! He is really terrified of me getting HG again as he feels he wouldn't cope looking after me, a toddler, the dog and the house all on his own and then be able to deal with a baby afterwards.*

(Anon, HG Survivor)

Socialising

This can be a tricky issue for couples who are perhaps used to socialising together. I (Caitlin) remember feeling extra alone and isolated when my husband would go to social engagements without me during my first pregnancy. It really compounded the misery, and I felt jealous of his ability to 'have a night off'. Even so, I knew at the time it was terribly unfair as he needed the break and I didn't want him to suffer just because I was suffering.

It is important you do take time off from caring. Perhaps try to arrange a friend or relative to come round to spend time with your partner while you go out to the pub or a party for a while. Be prepared for the potential fallout: as I explained above, it's not that she wants to withhold fun for you or make you suffer, rather it highlights her suffering and loneliness and the continuous nature of her condition.

Partner Chris Bloore explains how making time off for himself helped him support his wife better:

> *Make time for yourself. That's what worked for me. The thing that really wore me down was being on alert 24/7. If I was working at home, I had to be ready to sprint to the sofa with a sick bowl, water, a towel, pills, anything she may need. Taking an hour or two for myself, with no interruptions was invaluable. That time to me let me relax, unwind, and get ready to get back on alert. Take time for yourself once or twice a week, whatever you can both safely manage. If you can stay calm and happy, then you're much more effective than if you're tired and wound up all the time.*
>
> *It's okay to take time for yourself – it's really important. There was an article that my wife read in which a husband stated he knew his wife was really sick, but he was taking a beating too. As such, he needed to recover a bit as well. Once my wife read that, she was a little softer with me. Ultimately, you're going to have a baby. That's awesome. Never lose sight of that.*

But what is reasonable and what is not? Well, it will largely depend on the partnership you are in and your lifestyle and support network. Having been immersed in the HG world for some years, the authors of this book would advise that an evening at the pub or a friend's house is fine, as is a Saturday off, particularly if a friend or relative can stay with your partner. If you are both supposed to be at a wedding or event, then just you going may be acceptable if your partner is safe to be left for the duration. However, a lad's weekend away should probably be cancelled, and nipping out for a quick pint but returning at 3 a.m. steaming drunk is a definite no-no.

Now this may be a little controversial with the sufferers, but if your partner is admitted to hospital, then this is your opportunity for some respite. Visiting hours are usually over by 8 p.m. and not open again until 2 p.m. the next day. You know she is safe and being looked after so phone a friend and nip to the pub or bowling or the cinema, whatever you find relaxing. It will do you the world of good and refresh you for re-embracing the carer role on her return home. Women, if you are reading this too and disagree, then discuss your expectations with your partner.

Grow a Thick Skin

Easier said than done! As discussed earlier, the pregnancy hormones themselves can cause almighty and uncontrollable mood swings which women can find distressing. Hormones are so incredibly powerful – those of you who have witnessed a woman give birth and breast feed will be able to appreciate, all of that is done by hormones. In pregnancy, they literally control every aspect of your partner and are most likely the cause of the hyperemesis.

Make like a saint and don't rise to the snapping and shouting. Try to understand that she is suffering unimaginably, not just with the vomiting and nausea but with feelings of disappointment, guilt, anxiety, and potentially depression. We are all prone, whether pregnant or not, to lash out at those closest to us, so you are likely to be in the firing line quite often. Better to storm off for a short walk and come back calm than to say something you might later regret.

But if it's too late and you have said something cruel, then give yourself a break too, and when apologising, take the opportunity to talk to your partner about how hard you've been finding it watching her suffer and feeling so helpless. Let her know how much you wish you could share the burden of the sickness and remind her that it is only temporary.

> *They [the sufferers] lose a sense of self – everything they used to be able to do and enjoy is not possible. A simple walk down the road is not possible. They get depressed, short-tempered and take things out on you [the carer] and are hyper-critical despite your best efforts to support them. They don't mean to do it, it's just the illness.*
>
> *The hardest aspect of the pregnancy for me has been the way she takes a lot of sadness, irritation, and being fed up, out on me. She doesn't mean to, but there's no one else around.*

(Tom, HG Partner)

Asking for Help

This is something most people are really bad at. Society now is shaped by the nuclear family, and we are expected to get on with things and not moan too much. But actually, good friends and family members often really want to help. They just don't know how!

In my (Caitlin's) first pregnancy, when my husband used to go out without me, people would ask how I was and if there was anything they could do to help. When I realised he was naturally underplaying it, as we all do when things are tough, I realised I needed to send him out with a line. If anyone asked after me and how they can help he was to say, 'Actually, she's really lonely because she can't really get out of the house. She'd really love a visit!'. People would often respond with the fact that they had thought about popping by but were worried the time would be bad or I didn't want visitors. Suggest that they text her first so that if it's a bad time she can say so.

In my subsequent pregnancies, I learned very quickly that the help we really needed was around food and childcare. If people asked how they could help, I would happily inform them that if they could take Alfie (our first child) to the park next time they were going that would be really helpful. If they didn't have kids, then suggesting a meal for the freezer was generally met with welcome positivity. Friends with kids soon realised that offering dinner for my child, and perhaps husband too, really was a massive help and they were only too happy to oblige. I was able to rest in the quiet knowing that Alfie was having a wonderful time with his friends and was having a healthy family meal.

But you don't get if you don't ask! So swallow your pride, accept that you can't do everything because Superman doesn't actually exist. You are human.

Online Support

Women who have suffered hyperemesis commonly say that unless you have been through it, you simply can't understand what it's like. Partners report a similar phenomenon and find that other husbands/partners, whose wives had normal pregnancies without complications, just 'don't get it'. Therefore, online support for partners can be really great where you can connect with other partners who are supporting their loved one. It can be an opportunity to share tips and ideas for childcare help or managing your workload. It is also an opportunity to just mouth off about how hard it is for you. It is unlikely that anyone, even sufferers, will be able to appreciate this the way another partner/carer can.

There are opportunities on Facebook to hook up with other partners but safer and more effective is the forum on the PSS website. The details are in the appendix. If you register there, your partner will not be able to see your posts even if she is also registered. Equally you won't be able to see hers.

Employment Issues – Know Your Rights

Employees are entitled to time off for dealing with emergencies involving dependants such as children. This would cover a situation where a woman is taken into hospital and the partner needs to sort out childcare. You would be entitled to a reasonable amount of time off to deal with the emergency, for example, sorting out alternative childcare. But you would not be entitled to unlimited time off. There is no obligation on the employer to pay the employee in this situation but some choose to do so.

If you need more time off to look after children while your partner is unable then you might be eligible to take parental leave. Generally, the child must be under five, and this would be unpaid.

Under new law, no one can be discriminated against for issues related to pregnancy, even someone else's pregnancy. However, it is not unheard of for partners to lose their jobs over a hyperemesis pregnancy. If your job is at risk, you can seek help via Citizen's Advice. There are a number of links and resources in Appendix 1.

> *My husband has lost his job due to time away from the office taking me to hospital and caring for our daughter while I've been sick. We are in a legal dispute with them and have a strong case of pregnancy discrimination, but this has all added much unnecessary stress for us at what is already a very difficult time.*

(Abi, HG sufferer, UK)

Childcare – Know Your Options

You've got a few options in the United Kingdom for childcare, and if your wife is in hospital, it may be necessary for you to investigate them and make decisions. Even if older children are in school, you may need help outside of school hours and these will apply for them too.

1) A nursery – These can be quite pricey but offer a lot of flexibility with hours

as most are open 8 a.m. to 6 p.m. or even longer. So you may be able to fit drop off and pick-up around this or you may know other parents using the same nursery who could help with dropping off and picking up. Open all year and holiday time but generally closed over the Christmas period. They can usually provide food for children over 1 year old. But if your child is ill, they won't be able to go in or will be sent home if they get ill while there. If your child hasn't previously been in a nursery setting, then you may find they get ill an awful lot in the first few months.

2) A childminder – Often cheaper than nursery, some may not be as flexible with hours, whereas others will be more flexible. You will have to cope with the childminder having holidays, and if she is ill, you may have to find an alternative at very short notice. If your child is ill, they won't be able to go in either. The environment is often more 'homely' than a nursery though and routines can be more child-centred. A lot of childminders offer before and after school care for the school closest to them.

3) A nanny – This is a pricey option, and you will have administration to sort out such as insurance, tax, and so on (a link for a company that helps with this is in the appendix). But the benefits are huge, especially for the family dealing with hyperemesis. Nannies can be live in (in your house) or live out. Most nannies will cook for the children and do their washing as well as tidying and cleaning the areas the children use such as their bedrooms, bathroom, sitting room, and kitchen. If you work long or awkward hours, they can be very flexible, particularly if they live in. It could be reassuring to know there is an adult around if your partner is very ill at home too, and it's nice to have the one-to-one continuity for the children. If your kid is sick, the nanny still works, but if the nanny is sick, you may need to find an alternative at very short notice. To find a nanny going through an agency is often your best bet as they check references and can match you swiftly with an appropriate employee for your family but you may have to pay for the service or they may have a higher hourly rate than a privately sourced one. An agency will usually sort out employment contracts and so on for you and may be able to provide rapid short term sick cover if your nanny needs time off.

4) An au pair – is like a nanny but usually foreign, much cheaper and won't do as much in terms of hours and duties. Arranged through an agency, you

will need to provide free accommodation and food and pay around £200 per month minimum. You should be willing to treat them as part of the family and shouldn't rely too much on an au pair as part of the deal is they are here to learn English and usually attend college, but if you have school-aged children, this can be a great option for bridging the gap before and after school. If you have room in your house this is also a very cost effective solution for families that can afford or don't need a full time nanny.

5) Family and friends – There are rules about how much a friend can look after your child before they have to be registered as a childminder, but if grandparents are able to help out, then it is a very good option. Hopefully, free and flexible for awkward hours, but there are also drawbacks with it being tricky to broach things you're not happy with or if you want to change the situation.

Advocacy – Healthcare Professionals

It is very hard to advocate for oneself when you are barely able to speak for throwing up. HG can come on very suddenly and in a matter of days take a woman from the happiest moment of her life when she got a positive pregnancy test to the absolute worst moment of her life to date when she hasn't stopped being sick for days and is genuinely fearful for her life. It can change your once strong, confident, and articulate partner into someone unrecognisable and without any of those qualities.

It can be overwhelmingly scary and with such mixed emotions. Women can feel utterly lost and confused by what is happening – surely, this isn't 'normal morning sickness'. It's bad enough after a few days, but after weeks and weeks of unrelenting nausea and vomiting, few women have the strength to talk, let alone fight. Women may have been trying for months or even years to get pregnant only to be faced with feelings of devastation and guilt as fantasies of miscarriage or termination inevitably creep in.

And that is where partners can come in like knights in shining armour. Here are some tips about how to advocate for the hyperemesis sufferer.

Doctors can be kind of scary, can't they? If you are not from a medical background, then the chances are you look up to doctors and all their knowledge and have them on a bit of a pedestal. And rightly so – to a degree. They have been through years of education and training. They must be cleverer than the average person to have qualified, and they know a lot more than you about anatomy, physiology, pharmacology, how the NHS works, and so on. But they are not experts on everything. They can't be, they, like you, are human. And remembering that will help empower you to have a rational discussion with them.

So, following are some practical tips for advocating for your loved one:

1. Go in with a good attitude. Don't assume that the doctor will be dismissive, and don't assume that you will have to 'fight' for treatment. If you are reasonable, then they will have a hard time explaining why they are being unreasonable.

2. Prepare yourself in advance. Take notes in with you, in particular about her symptoms, your concerns, and any questions.

Symptoms:	How many times a day is she vomiting? How much fluid and food has she kept down in 24/hours? How often is she passing urine? Has she lost much weight? If she can't get down the stairs for dizziness and vomiting, then note that down. Is movement, sound, and smell triggering vomiting?
Your concerns:	What are your main worries? That she is severely dehydrated? That she has lost so much weight? That she is bed-bound and getting sores or at risk of DVT? That if you leave her alone to go to work she may fall down the stairs because she is so dizzy and weak? That you are both going to lose your jobs over this?
Questions:	Is it safer to take medication or not? If she is not being admitted now, then at what point should you be concerned that she needs to go to hospital? What signs and symptoms should you look out for that things are more serious? What is the best route for speaking to the GP, can you email or phone to speak to them? Could you help by monitoring her ketones at home? Could the nurse teach you to give her intramuscular injections of her medications for times that she can't manage oral ones? Is there any other support you can get with this?

3. When you first go in, explain that your partner is finding it difficult to speak due to the symptoms and you would like to explain what's been going on on her behalf. If the doctor seems put out by that, then go on to explain that just getting to the surgery has been a real struggle and she really would prefer you did the talking. The doctor can always confirm that with your partner if they want.

4. Using your notes as above explain that while you were both prepared for a bit of 'morning sickness' and know it's a normal part of pregnancy, you really don't think this severity is normal and you think she has hyperemesis gravidarum. Explain that whilst you had hoped to have a nice natural pregnancy, without medication and so on, you really feel that she needs some treatment as the symptoms are so severe. You under stand they aren't licensed for pregnancy but feel that when looked at from a risk/benefit perspective, you both think the time has come to accept that she needs treatment.

5. Now assuming your doctor has reacted really well and is being kind and proactive, ask for a plan going forward. He doesn't need to agree to more medication or anything else yet if it is not deemed necessary, but he does need to let you know what symptom severity to look out for and when to come back if things don't improve. If he is sending you home rather than hospital, then ask what he would like you to monitor, that is, fluid intake/output, ketones (he can prescribe Ketostix or you can buy them online or at chemists). Ask him what his criteria are for needing treatment.

Hopefully, by following these steps, you will develop a good working relationship with your GP and feel that you have managed to help your loved one by getting her treatment and support. But what if it doesn't go to plan as above? What if despite your careful description of her symptoms and your concerns, the doctor still fobs you off with 'it's normal' or 'no medication is safe in pregnancy'.

Well, if the doctor is trying to claim it is normal, then ask at what point they would consider severe nausea and vomiting to not be normal and what level of dehydration they consider acceptable for a pregnant woman.

If they give you and your partner a hard time about taking medication in pregnancy and claim it isn't safe and you might be damaging the baby, then ask for the evidence base for such claims. Point out that there is more evidence that not treating hyperemesis effectively has risks for the baby and mother than treating with medications for which there is no evidence of adverse foetal outcomes (you might want to write that down).

Remember that GPs generally don't know what the next patient to walk through the door is suffering with until they sit down and tell them. HG is not particularly common with many GPs seeing only one or two cases a year and they can't keep up to date with all of the research about every condition. So try to be sympathetic to that, perhaps signpost them to the PSS charity pages about treatments and perhaps offer to give them some time to look into the options, you could phone back in the afternoon or pick a prescription up later.

Recognise too that getting the treatment right can be a case of trial and error, so always ask for advice on how long to give the medication to work and what to do if there is no improvement or she gets side effects or her condition deteriorates. Doctors can feel frustrated if a patient is expecting a cure from them when there is no cure to give. Accepting that there is no cure, yet, and that you need to look to 'manage' the condition will help no end.

The aim of the game is to build up a "team feeling" with your doctor; make it clear you want to work with them to help your partner, you are all on the same side and don't expect a quick solution from them.

Ultimately though, if you don't feel you've been treated well or got the help you need, then ask to see someone else. Go out to reception and ask for another appointment with someone else. If you have the strength and feel you have grounds, you could ask to speak to the practice manager or make a complaint. But keep it in perspective. Getting help for your partner needs to come first. Remember you are entitled to change practice surgery to see a different set of doctors and you can contact Pregnancy Sickness Support to find out if they know of any 'HG Friendly' doctors in your area.

Other HCPs you may find yourself having to speak to on behalf of your wife are nurses and midwives. You are unlikely to need to discuss treatments with them, but you may find yourself defending her against ignorant comments. Sometimes it's just not worth it –

> *During my 12 week scan with my third HG pregnancy, the midwife sonographer subjected me to a lecture about the cure for hyperemesis. It was all about diet and eating little and often. I made a couple of feeble attempts to explain that eating little and often was only possible if you could keep a*

little down, then I gave up – it simply wasn't worth it. I mean, what did she think? That I was munching three big meals everyday? My husband was trying not to laugh at this midwife as he knew I was working, as a trustee, on the development of the PSS website at the time, had read vast amounts of research on HG, and knew far more about the condition than she ever would. We left the room and although I was fuming we joked about the 'crackering' we had just received. In that case, being able to laugh together was great. In my first pregnancy, I would have left in tears wishing my husband could have spoken up for me. Remember – pick your battles!

(Caitlin, Author)

Advocating with Friends and Work Colleagues

I shall start this how the last paragraph was left off – Pick your battles! Some people simply cannot change their narrow-minded view and trying to make them only ends in you feeling frustrated and angry.

That said, the authors of this book are all about raising awareness about hyperemesis and would encourage everyone to speak up about the reality of it.

You will hear hurtful comments from people who mean well and some people who don't mean so well. Women get terribly frustrated hearing comments about thinking positively and getting some fresh air or trying ginger. But it's frustrating for the partners too. Paradoxically though if a partner of a sufferer were to correct a person's ignorant comment with a swift retort, it is likely to have a much more powerful impact than coming from the sufferer herself. Here are a couple to try for some of the more classic comments you are likely to encounter:

- 'If we could have avoided all the medication and IV drips with ginger, we definitely would have, sadly it's not that simple'
- 'My wife is a very positive person, but you can't "think better" a broken leg and you can't "think better" hyperemesis'
- 'Eating little and often is very effective for mild to moderate pregnancy sickness, but if you can't keep anything down at all, it's not much use'
- 'It sounds like your wife had morning sickness, that's not what my wife has. It's a severe complication of pregnancy called hyperemesis, and before IV

drips and modern medicine, it was the leading cause of death in early pregnancy – I'm grateful she is still alive!'

Speaking to employers on her behalf can be useful as it demonstrates just how ill she is if she can't even speak on the phone. If she is having problems with work, then you need to look up about her rights and take control of the situation for her. In the United Kingdom, a woman cannot be discriminated against because of a pregnancy-related condition. There is information on the PSS website about employment rights in relation to pregnancy sickness, and there are other links and contacts in the appendix.

As her advocate and partner, you need to feel empowered to speak and act on her behalf. Take the responsibility seriously and have confidence in your ability to do so – you will be helping her so much by taking charge of these issues for her and defending her rights. Polish up that shiny knight's armour in your head and picture yourself with a sword and big shield.

While researching to write this book, we spoke to a number of partners of sufferers about what they wanted to see in here. A number of men said they would really like to know what not to say. So here is a list of the main hyperemesis faux pas for while she is being sick, and what she will be thinking if you say them:

1. *Can you keep the noise down?* Er no!
2. *Ew! The cornflakes look just the same as before you ate them* – Gee, thanks for the commentary!
3. *Wow, that sick really stinks* – If emptying my sick bowl by all means think it, just don't say it!
4. *Better out than in* – not helpful, particularly when nothing has stayed in for weeks and behind the constant nausea is a feeling of constant hunger!
5. *Well, that's put me off my lunch* – Oh boo hoo for you!
6. *I thought you said you hadn't eaten anything?* – Ouch, a touch of the not believing! Not just the wrong thing to say but outright nasty.
7. *You ought to be used to it by now* – Hmmm... How about I keep hitting you with a stick and see if you get used to it?

8. *Did you spill some water?* – Er no, but you've just added to my humiliation.

9. *Don't puke the baby up!* – Yeah I know you're trying to be funny but it's really not!

10. *Well – you wanted this pregnancy* – ouch! Yeah I wanted a pregnancy but I never asked for HG!

And here is a list you may want to copy and provide to family and friends, before they visit or phone, of what not to say:

1. *'Have you tried ginger?'* This has got to be the all-time greatest thing not to say. Research has found that all women with any level of pregnancy sickness know about the 'taking ginger' remedy. What most people don't know (although plenty of veteran HG sufferers do) is that the only form of ginger which has found to be in any way helpful is as a capsule, 1,000 mg per day and then it is only helpful for mild queasiness. Ginger biscuits, ginger ale, ginger tea, ginger ice lollies... it's all old wives' tales. Do you really think a woman who is on powerful anti-emetics and IV fluids could really have avoided all that suffering if she had only tried a bit of ginger? Furthermore, side effects include painful heartburn and potential issues with blood clotting.

2. *'Oh I had that, but I still went to work and got on with life'*. Well, then you didn't! that is like comparing a twisted ankle to a broken leg.

3. '*Think positively and get some fresh air*' By saying this, it implies that it is all in her mind and she is causing her own suffering. It's a terribly cruel thing to say and a sure-fired way to lose a friend.

4. *'Well, at least you can get pregnant... you should be grateful for that'*. We know and we are. Pointing it out just adds to the guilt the woman is already inevitably experiencing due to feeling negative towards the pregn ancy and for 'not feeling grateful'. It cuts deep and the pain lasts. Plenty of women with hyperemesis have even been through the pain of experiencing both and are pregnant thanks to IVF, so the hurt for them is all the more.

5. *'I loved every moment of pregnancy. It's such a special time, creating life, glowing blah blah blah blah'.* Well, bully for you and thanks for rubbing my nose in my misery!

6. *'Is it safe to be taking those drugs? Won't they harm the baby?'*. No wom an actually wants to take medication in pregnancy. We all (well most) go into pregnancy wanting to be natural earth mothers eating healthy and avoiding all potential harm. Sadly, some women cannot survive pregnancy without medication. In the past, before the invention of modern medicine, women would simply die. Often without knowing why as symptoms would kill her before a pregnancy was confirmed or even suspected. Women with HG taking medication think dozens of times everyday about the safety of the medication, questioning if they really need them and if the baby will be okay, but the reality is the drugs are prescribed by a doctor and given because they are needed. They are ultimately much safer than not taking them. As little as we know about the specific effects of the medication, we also know little about the effects of severe dehydration, a baby bathed in ketones and a malnourished mum. To add to her concern and worry and to make her feel like she needs to justify her condition is wrong and actually really inappropriate. If a pregnant woman was having an asthma attack, would you question if the steroid inhaler was safe? No, you'd be pumping away worried that she may die without it!

The next chapter is specifically for family and friends, and you are welcome to photocopy the pages for them or you can download information for them from the Spewing Mummy website.

Mental Health – the Issues and What To Do If You're Worried

Back in the 1930s, around the time of psychodynamic theory development, the mad, excuse the pun, idea developed that women with HG were mentally ill and that the excessive, life-threatening vomiting was down to a subconscious rejection of the foetus or a symptom of an unhappy marriage. This coincided with a drop in the death rate from the condition, thanks to the incredibly wonderful development of intravenous fluids. But not dying combined with ridiculous theories about women's mental states led to abominable treatment plans where women were literally locked up, prevented from seeing family, and left to rot in their own vomit having had sick bowls removed and nurses told not to help them clean up.

Thankfully, on the whole, that kind of stuff doesn't happen any more, although due to staff shortages, it isn't uncommon for women in hospital to have to dispose of their own vomit bowls.

Even more thankfully, the idea of a psychological cause has been utterly disproved.

However, there can be no denying that HG can cause mental health issues for the sufferer. The prolonged suffering of continuous, unrelenting nausea and vomiting, vomiting which in itself can be violent, painful, and unpredictable, takes a massive toll. The isolation of literally months in bed with only minutes a day of company from a partner who is at work the rest of the time or caring for other children can be immense. Unable to read, speak on the phone, watch TV, or gain any respite from focusing on the crippling nausea makes the time seem to pass even slower. And the humiliation that comes when vomiting results in urinating on the floor or in your bed or the knowledge you haven't showered in weeks all adds to the overall mental toll on your partner – it's hardly any wonder depression can ensue.

Perinatal (during pregnancy) depression is not uncommon. I (Caitlin) was certainly depressed during pregnancy as a direct result of HG. I was lucky though that it didn't last beyond pregnancy because for many women, perinatal depression leads to postnatal depression and that can be far more serious than many people realise – ultimately, for some it can be fatal. It is also important to monitor your own mental health. Amanda's husband suffered from depression following her pregnancy, and it is easy to see how this can happen when you consider the trauma you both go through during a hyperemesis pregnancy. But it can be so easy to forget your own health when focussing so much on supporting your partner through it!

Post Traumatic Stress Disorder (PTSD) can also be common after a hyperemesis pregnancy. It's hardly surprising if you look at the causes of the condition – prolonged exposure to an extremely stressful situation. Well, lying in bed for weeks or months vomiting on every movement and thinking you are dying is pretty stressful. Flashbacks are common with this, as is emetophobia (fear of vomiting) and food or pregnancy-related anxiety and panic attacks. PTSD too can be terminal and should never be underestimated.

Luckily though, these conditions are treatable, and the first thing you must do if you think your partner is suffering is to talk to her about getting help. Then get help! Don't just ignore it and hope she'll get better and don't assume she will get help for herself. Express your concerns, but if you are met with resistance and denial, then don't be put of getting help for her.

In Appendix 1, there are some links to organisations that may be able to help. If your GP or midwife were helpful during the pregnancy, then you could try them for a referral to a local service. Postnatal depression tends to be well recognised and supported these days and you will hopefully be met with empathy and kindness if you seek help for this. Unfortunately though, peri-natal depression and HG-related PTSD tend to be a little less recognised. It's improving, but if your first attempt to get help fails, then try, try, and try again using the avenues in the appendix. If your partner wants you to advocate for her and go with her to the doctor, then do and use the same techniques as outlined earlier in the chapter. But above all, get help. It's bad enough she suffered in pregnancy – don't let the legacy of HG ruin any more of your lives – take control and get help!

Don't Suffer in Silence – Get Help!

For easy reference, here is a list of symptoms which may raise alarm bells for you and could be used as a way of talking to your partner about your concerns:

- Continuous low mood or sadness
- Feeling of hopelessness and helplessness
- Low self-esteem
- Tearfulness
- Feelings of guilt
- Feeling irritable and intolerant of others
- Lack of motivation and little interest in things
- Difficulty making decisions
- Lack of enjoyment
- Suicidal thoughts or thoughts of harming someone else
- Feeling anxious or worried
- Change in appetite or weight (outside normal post-pregnancy/post-hyperemesis)

- Lack of energy or lack of interest in sex (outside normal new parent exhaustion)
- Disturbed sleep patterns and insomnia
- Taking part in fewer social activities and avoiding contact with friends
- Reduced hobbies and interests

This list is not exhaustive and further information is available online.

Conclusion

Hyperemesis is an illness that can have a profound effect on the partner of the sufferer. Support and care of your loved one is a challenge and can be utterly exhausting, but recognising you are in this together and fostering a team attitude to surviving will help you both.

We hope this chapter has offered some practical tips and advice on what you can do to support your partner and to get through the ordeal yourself. There are various avenues to explore for help and support and you do not have to face this alone.

> *If anyone says they are always empathetic and can give unlimited amounts of sympathy, love, support, and understanding, they are lying. Eventually it wears a little thin. That's when you need to remove yourself for a bit go for a walk, put some headphones on for an hour, give yourself a little time, and go back again with a refreshed aspect.*

(Tom, HG Partner)

CHAPTER 8

Tips for Family and Friends

Under no circumstances mention the phrase, 'Have you tried ginger?' or 'I hear ginger helps' or 'being sick is a good sign, means it's a healthy pregnancy'. It's no help whatsoever to the HG sufferer!

(Pauline, HG sufferer)

Watching a loved one suffer with NVP or HG can be really tough, and it can be harder still to know how best to help and support them. Trying to appreciate and understand what they are going through is the first step in trying to help and support her.

Never visit a person with hyperemesis and say you had morning sickness so you know what they are going through! It is not morning sickness!–

(Sarah, HG sufferer)

The reality is that no one intentionally hurts or upsets a friend who is suffering. They simply don't realise the impact their innocent, well-meaning suggestions can have. Often people feel very out of their depth trying to help a friend who is suffering in a way they can't personally imagine. And why should we be able to understand an experience which we haven't been through? Some things we can imagine are universally horrendous for anyone (deaths of loved ones and so on) but of ailments, which we have no personal experience, how are we meant to know?

The hip pain at night during pregnancy was awful, but I honestly can't imagine what symphysis pubis dysfunction (SPD) is like because I didn't have it. To have that pain constantly! The GP who gave me such excellent and compassionate care never had any pregnancy sickness, but she did have terrible SPD and described it as 'every step was agony, like walking on broken glass, and no-one understood'.

Had I not have suffered HG myself, I would have been the first to suggest the alternative remedies for pregnancy sickness, SPD, and any other pregnancy aliment which I would assume myself to be an expert on simply from having been pregnant myself. Now I try to relay my experience with one misunderstood condition and apply similar sensitivity to other people's misunderstood conditions such as SPD, migraine, myalgic encephalomyelitis, fibromyalgia, depression, and so on.

(Caitlin, Author)

So here are a few ways you can offer support to your friend or relative while she is suffering:

- Just listen and believe her. Unfortunately, no suggestions you make are going to miraculously cure the HG and not suggesting them won't make her think you don't care. Quite the opposite! By not suggesting those things, which she will already have heard so many times before, she will enjoy your company and support all the more.
- Offer practical support such as making some meals for the freezer that her partner will appreciate too, but please don't put any garlic in it... her partner won't appreciate relegation to the spare room for stinking!
- When visiting, make your own cup of tea and wash up your mug (along with any other dishes lying around) before you leave.
- If she already has kids, then perhaps take them out for the day. She'll be comforted to know they are having fun with friends and they will enjoy some carefree time with non-parental adults.
- Going to the supermarket? Text to ask if she needs any essentials, bread, milk, etc. If you drop them over, put them in the fridge for her. A lot of women with hyperemesis can't stand the smell of the fridge.
- Be sensitive to how strong her sense of smell is. It's not just strong, but it's warped too, so once pleasant smells are absolutely revolting. Therefore, if visiting, avoid strong perfume, eating garlic the night before, smoking prior to visit, and so on. As nice as flowers are she is likely not able to toler ate the smell.
- If you want to get her gifts, then remember that chocolates are a no-no unless she has specified wanting them. A magazine would be better, perhaps rather than a pregnancy or girly one how about something that interests her like countryside, knitting, photography, etc. Explain that while you appreciate she can't do those things at the moment, you hoped that she would be able to flick through the pictures during her better moments

and distract herself a little. Other thoughtful gifts would be some comfort able pyjamas or slippers, audiobooks, or a new cushion.

- While you are visiting, nip to the loo and give it a clean. Don't tell her you're going to do that or ask if she wants you to... who on earth would say, 'Yes, please, if you don't mind cleaning the splatters of vomit off the inside of my toilet, I'd really appreciate it'?

- Send her texts to check up on her and let her know you are thinking of her, but don't get offended if she doesn't reply all the time or with any speed. Phone screen–induced vomiting is pretty standard but so too is the loneliness and depression which makes you want to shut off from the whole world, especially those who have never suffered. Your texts will mean more to her than you can imagine.

- If her partner works and isn't able to attend doctor appointments and you are able to go with her, then great, advocate for her. If she can't speak for herself, then speak up on her behalf. Tell the doctor or midwife how it really is. She's not being sick in a normal way two to three times a day; it's relent less, x–y times per day. She may not have the strength herself. There is more information on advocacy in the partner's section.

- If she is worried about prescribed medications, then do a bit of research to reassure her of the safety – Contact the charity PSS for more info or the HER Foundation outside the United Kingdom.

A lot of those things may seem quite demanding of your time and energy and perhaps difficult to fit into a busy life with children and work. A lot of it will depend on how good a friend you are and the personal circumstances – a sister is likely going to do more than a work colleague. But if you aim for the above and avoid unhelpful comments (see also chapter 7 for more details, the partner's section), then you're on your way to winning the award for Best Friend of the Year!

If she seems to be shutting herself off from you, refusing visits, and not calling, then try to remember that vomiting in front of people can be really humiliating and she may be scared of seeing people in case she is sick. Or she may just not have the energy. At its worst, hyperemesis can reduce a woman to a state of lying still with vomit trickling from her mouth as she retches every few minutes. Many women experience ptyalism (excessive saliva production) which can be embarrassing, and later on in pregnancy, vomiting can result in episodes of urinary incontinence. All of these can put women off from wanting to see even their very best friends. Don't be disheartened if she seems to be avoiding you. Just text regularly to remind her you are there for her and are thinking of her. It's a nice feeling to know you are missed by your friends, and she will gain comfort knowing you are there even if she doesn't feel up to seeing you.

Bear in mind also that a number of the medications used to treat hyperemesis can cause drowsiness and other side effects. So even if you do go round to visit and she doesn't seem chatty or looks like she is nodding off, don't take it personally. Remember she is very ill and medicated. Encourage her to rest. If she already has a child at home, then as much as you wanted to see her, it would be far more helpful if she could go for a nap while you watch her children.

If, however, when you visit, you become concerned that she is very dehydrated (dry lips and tongue, dry skin, etc) or she seems unusually confused or drowsy, then call her doctor or take her to hospital. Dehydration can become rapidly serious, and because of confusion that it causes, it's not uncommon for women to accidentally take too many doses of anti-emetics or other medications.

Regardless of how bad the woman is suffering and, to be honest, what the condition is (I'm sure the above would apply to plenty of acute and chronic illnesses: cancer, flu, depression, broken limbs, etc.), ultimately a bit of compassion goes a long way and is often appreciated all the more if it's acknowledged that you can't actually imagine the suffering they are experiencing but you want to help if you can.

Here are some quick dos and don'ts for visiting times:

DO

- Offer to pick up any shopping or prescriptions on your way round.
- Bring some magazines and books (but bear in mind she may not be up to reading/watching) – Downloading some audiobooks for her could be really wonderful!
- If you go to the loo, give it a quick clean... there is not much worse than vomiting into an unclean toilet!

- If she is largely bed-bound, then offer to change/wash the bedspreads for her.
- If you put any washing on for her, don't use scented fabric softener.
- If she is struggling with young children, then offer to play with them while she has a lie down. Bring quiet activities to occupy them at other times.
- Make sure you wash any mugs or pots before you leave.
- Just listen to her, rather than trying to make suggestions.

DON'T

- Wear perfume.
- Eat garlic or curry the night before a visit.
- Smoke before visiting.
- Quiz her on her medication and what she is doing to 'help herself'
- Bring flowers as a gift; as well meaning as they are, the smell and colours can trigger vomiting. (Silk flowers are fine and a nice reminder of your friendship and support for years to come)
- Expect her to make tea and coffee, make it yourself!
- Bring noisy children with you.
- Focus on the pregnancy or the illness; try to talk about 'normal' things.
- Leave any mess for her to clear up!

CHAPTER 9

Ending the Hyperemesis Pregnancy – Termination

Around 10% of wanted pregnancies complicated by hyperemesis end in termination, and of them, very few have been offered the full range of treatments available. We don't have a statistic for how many women consider or think about terminating their pregnancy, but based on the experience of PSS staff who are dealing daily with hyperemesis sufferers, the number is massive. So you are definitely not alone if you are confused by thoughts about terminating a baby you tried for, many of us have been there.

Plenty of terminations happen regardless of hyperemesis, and that is the woman's choice and she is entitled to access a safe and supportive service with non-judgemental advice from HCPs. In these cases, she should not be denied treatment for hyperemesis simply because she is ending the pregnancy. In fact, quite the opposite, treatment of symptoms should be forthcoming. However, we are assuming if you are reading this book, it is because you planned your baby and want to keep it (or didn't plan it but still want to keep it) and the chapter continues with this assumption.

Most cases of termination for hyperemesis are avoidable with proper treatment and support. However, far too often ineffective or inadequate care leaves women feeling they have no option but to terminate their wanted pregnancy.

> *My husband actually printed off information about ondansetron and steroid treatment and we begged the doctors to let us try them before terminating. But they refused and said they weren't safe for the baby. So we terminated. We had no choice. I regretted it straight away. How can medication be less safe for the baby than termination? –*

(Anon, HG Sufferer, who went on to survive hyperemesis the following year and now has a baby)

Early intervention with effective medications can often prevent the need for termination. However, as we have discussed earlier in this book, many doctors are nervous about prescribing anti-emetics, particularly in early pregnancy.

Women who are left untreated or in rare, extreme cases, who don't respond to the treatments in current use can become seriously ill. Metabolic imbalances, organ failure, or complications from treatments such as PICC lines can mean that a therapeutic termination is required to save the mother's life. If you are in this situation and your doctors are recommending a termination due to severe complications, you may have no choice in the matter and saving your life should take priority.

These cases are very rare though, and generally, termination should be considered as a treatment only as a last resort after all other treatment options have been exhausted. If you have just got this book and turned straight to this section because you are at the point of considering this, then please turn back to the section about treatments. Then get in touch with the charities listed in the appendix for support and the most up-to-date treatment. They can also put you in touch with 'HG Friendly' doctors in your area who should be willing to try the full range of treatments before considering termination.

> *It was horrific. This was a very much wanted pregnancy. I was so desperate though, I had absolutely no choice. My care had been so bad the hyperemesis had spiralled totally out of control. I was alone in a hospital bed for weeks, hardly seeing anyone unless bags of fluid needed changing or drugs administering. I couldn't even cuddle my husband as his smell made me feel sick (he smells great by the way!) I swear I could smell the baby coming through my skin. I begged them to take me to theatre that night, and that I wouldn't hold it against them. I told them what they wanted to hear so they would agree. Afterwards I was recovered fine, no more sickness. I still feel angry but I don't feel guilty. I know that sounds awful but I know I must have been at rock-bottom, at my wits' end, to have made that decision for such a wanted baby. This is how I deal with what I did.*

(Anon, HG Survivor)

Termination is not an easy option and is not without risks, although these are often skimmed over and underestimated. The lasting physiological and psychological effects can be severe and can be worse with repeated terminations. The trauma and grief from terminating a wanted, even tried for baby can take a lot of time and healing to recover from. You should seek help with this process.

In terms of what a termination involves, it depends on the stage of pregnancy. Before about 9 weeks, there is the option of a medical termination, but beyond this point, a termination involves a surgical procedure. It is beyond the scope of this book to go into details about the procedures, but organisations such as Marie Stopes provide extensive information on their website and at their centres. Contact details of these organisations are in Appendix 1, so you can contact them for further information. You can also ask your GP for information, advice, and a referral.

If you have been through a termination because of hyperemesis and are now considering trying again, then there are post-termination counselling services you can get in touch with. If you decide you do want to try again after a termination, then planning your next pregnancy is going to be key and your doctors should be willing to be pro-active and involved in the planning stage. Judgement and personal opinion on a woman's choice has no place in the medical profession, and if you are faced with a GP treating you harshly because of this, you have the right to see another doctor – you would also have grounds for complaint. It is terribly sad that in this day and age, women are still faced with attitudes like this, although thankfully they are becoming rarer.

Here are some stories from women who have been through termination for hyperemesis. Our aim by sharing these is not to scare or upset women in this situation or who have been through termination themselves. Rather we hope to let women know they are not alone and also demonstrate how in almost every case it is a lack of treatment which results in termination. All of these stories are kept anonymous.

> *After a terrible HG pregnancy, I was terrified when I got pregnant again. Not knowing about the treatments available for hyperemesis, I went to my GP and we discussed terminating. Rather than looking at the treatments available, she did the referral without question and refused to prescribe any anti-sickness medication in the meantime. 'In case you change your mind and the medication harmed the baby,' she said. I was terrified. I thought I might die this time and I already had a baby that needed me. I didn't want him to grow up without a mum. No one told me there were safe treatments I could have tried.*

> *My husband printed off research about using ondansetron and steroids and how safe they are, but the doctors wouldn't read it. They said they couldn't prescribe them. They told me that I had ketones in my urine and*

that meant my organs were failing and I might die if I don't terminate, so I did. I didn't have a choice... I didn't want to die. I found out after when I joined a support group that ketones doesn't mean my organs are failing. They never even took a blood test. Lots of other women in this country take ondansetron and steroids, but they wouldn't let me try them.

The real medical details are hazy as I was so poorly and to be honest have blocked it out I think, but I'll tell you what I remember. I did not even know HG existed and no one ever told me that was what I had. I was not even offered any medication even though I asked for some anti-emetics and was told they were not suitable for pregnancy. I don't remember who first mentioned termination, but once it was suggested, I begged for it (I think I was about 8 weeks) and was very judgementally given the go ahead for one. Only then was I prescribed metoclopramide (with the warning that even then she was reluctant to hand them out as I may change my mind). The tablets did not work. My symptoms actually got worse on them. I was also made to wait a very long time for my termination, and I was about 13 weeks when I had it and it was very traumatic. That was 3 years ago, and only recently, I have been able to grieve for my baby. We tried again the following year, and as soon as I was pregnant, the HG kicked in (earlier and nastier this time). I went to the same GP, but she refused to see me. I was still not given anti-emetics (I didn't know about options available). I arranged an early booking in appointment with the midwife, but it was horrendous – she shouted at me for bothering to book in early and told me I just had morning sickness and to eat fruit and drink water – despite vomiting non-stop for over a week. On a telephone consult, the GP refused to talk to me and had me passed onto a locum GP. When I asked what I could do as I was so ill, he demanded to know 'if I wanted to keep this baby'. I was admitted to hospital the next day in a wheelchair because I was too weak to walk. Still I only got cyclizine and metoclopramide, and domperidone and spent the whole of my pregnancy fighting to get through every day. I'm suffering with PTSD now, and I am currently very angry that I had never even heard of ondansetron until I joined an online support group last year. How on earth are people supposed to know that that level of sickness is not normal and that there is hope out there if doctors just brush you off?'

I fell pregnant in early 2012. My baby was 6 months old, and it was a tremendous shock because I was on contraception and I suffer with hyperemesis, so I would be unable to care for my baby should I become ill. Last time it hadn't started so early, but this time, the hyperemesis set in straight away. I knew I was pregnant without doing the test, but as soon as I did a test and it was positive, I immediately called my doctor. I explained the situation and begged for ondansetron or steroids because I knew about these and had read research about them. I explained that there was no way I could care for my baby and have sickness especially at the severity that it was during my last pregnancy. I was totally bedridden and suffered severe weight loss and depression. The doctor refused to prescribe steroids and wouldn't even discuss ondansetron. She would only prescribe the first-line anti-emetic, which hadn't helped me last time. She said if I get ill enough, I would have to go to hospital. In my desperation, I said, 'Well, I am going to have to terminate,' because I hoped that she would prescribe me medication if she understood how desperate I was. The doctor said that she didn't see any other option for me in my current situation as I had no one to care for my young baby should I be very ill. At this point I was really scared. The HG worsened over days, and I was unable to hold down even a sip of water, at least with my previous pregnancy I had been able to sip water. I actually got scared that I might die. My mother had to look after my child full-time during the weeks that I tried to battle through it as my husband had to work, but eventually, she had to return to work and my sickness medication wasn't helping. In fact, it was getting worse and worse. I contacted BPAS and waited a further 2 weeks for a termination. I was 10 weeks pregnant when I terminated. No one asked if I had tried all the alternatives, and I was never referred to a consultant; I was too ill to fight for these things and I didn't know how to. I have suffered with mental health problems since the termination; it was very traumatic. We are trying to accept that we can't have any more children, but it's not easy.

Part III

Life After Hyperemesis

CHAPTER 10

Getting Back to 'Normal'

One of the things that runs through your mind when you are suffering from relentless nausea and/or daily bouts of vomiting is whether you will ever feel 'normal' again. It can be hard to even remember what 'normal' feels like when every day is spent lying in bed trying not to vomit and desperately hoping that at some point this awful sickness is going to go away. It becomes your constant companion, the one thing that never fails to turn up day after day, and you can find it hard to remember what it felt like not to be nauseous all the time. And this may lead to the worry that this sickness may never end, not even when the pregnancy is over.

But be assured it will end and you will, once again, find yourself free of nausea. Some women say that the sickness disappears almost instantly as soon as the placenta is delivered; others report a lingering sense of nausea and the odd bout of vomiting that occur just after they have given birth. Ultimately, HG ends once the pregnancy is over. It just may take a little bit longer for some than others.

That being said, some women do report symptoms post-pregnancy that they never suffered from before and severe HG can take time to recover from. The authors have found that certain health issues are discussed frequently amongst women who have had a HG pregnancy, and it is these issues that we will focus on in this chapter. However, as with any condition, there is always the risk of other conditions being developed at the same time purely by coincidence, and it can be very hard to separate the two and very easy to blame the hyperemesis for everything thereafter.

Therefore, before we go any further, it is important to note that what is 'normal' for one person may be completely abnormal for another. We cannot define what normal is for any one person and so if you are worried about any symptoms that develop during or after your pregnancy please do see your GP to discuss these. Likewise, we cannot define what 'getting back to normal' means as even after a pregnancy without HG issues can arise which are far from 'normal' for that woman. As always, use this book as a guide only and always speak to your own GP about any concerns you have, whether they are ongoing symptoms or new problems.

So let's look at the most frequently discussed issues that women talk about following a HG pregnancy:

Reflux

Acid reflux and indigestion seem to be fairly common issues following a HG pregnancy, even in women who never had a problem with this prior to pregnancy. It may have been a major issue during the pregnancy itself and you may have been looking forward to the day when you could eat and drink whatever you liked without suffering from the pain and nausea which can accompany acid reflux. And for some women the problem ends with the end of the pregnancy, but for others it may continue, much to their dismay.

The good news is that, generally speaking, the reflux will not be anywhere near as severe as it was during pregnancy, especially during the third trimester when reflux becomes an unpleasant and persistent problem even for women without HG. Although eating pretty much anything during pregnancy can lead to painful reflux, it's often certain triggers post-pregnancy that cause it. Triggers could include certain foods, particularly sweet or fatty foods, or jumping up straight after eating, which realistically happens a lot once you have a little one to chase after! Finding what works best to help you deal with this issue will depend on your own situation.

Your GP can describe medication to help control the symptoms of reflux and so if you are having ongoing issues with it and over-the-counter products are not quite cutting it then do go and speak to your GP, particularly if symptoms are persisting for months after pregnancy or are getting worse. In these cases your doctor may need to investigate further to see if there is an underlying issue (such as a hiatus hernia), which may affect the choice of treatment chosen to control symptoms and without treatment can lead to further complications.

In the short term, reducing your intake of fatty, fried, sugary and spicy foods may help reduce symptoms and sleeping a little propped up can reduce night time symptoms. Further self help can be found on NHS websites such as NHS Choices.

Nausea, Especially During the Latter Part of the Menstrual Cycle

Another relatively common discussion the authors have seen on HG forums is that of nausea and/or vomiting during the menstrual cycle. For some women, this may be a heightened degree of nausea compared to what they experienced pre-pregnancy, but for others, it can be a totally new experience.

The nausea and/or vomiting are generally experienced in the latter part of the menstrual cycle, usually around the time the period starts. However, for some, the symptoms could start as early as ovulation and continue until the bleeding begins. The intensity of symptoms varies from woman to woman, with some having full-blown HG-like symptoms for a day or so whilst others experience more manageable levels of nausea. No matter what degree of intensity the symptoms are, they are still a very unpleasant and often distressing reminder of the many weeks and months of HG symptoms and can even leave some women convinced they must have fallen pregnant to be experiencing such symptoms again.

Just like with HG, the reason behind these symptoms is unknown, and it can be frustrating to suffer from them each month. And again, as with HG, the best way of treating it varies from woman to woman. Hormonal contraceptives and anti-emetics may be prescribed, and it may take some time to find the right solution for you. Your decision regarding hormonal contraceptives will depend on if and when you plan to try for another baby. For instance, a Mirena coil is great for people wanting something to last several years but not so good for someone wanting to try to conceive several months down the line. Your GP or Practice Nurse will be able to discuss all your options with you.

Cyclical Vomiting Syndrome (CVS) is a condition in its own right, and if ongoing nausea and/or vomiting is an issue for you, this may be something that needs addressing. It is beyond the scope of this book to address it though. There is no known link between CVS and HG, but by the very nature of coincidence, there are likely to be a number of unlucky women who will suffer both conditions, and it is hard not to assume a link if you are one of them.

Incontinence and Piles

Unlike the two issues above, incontinence and piles are actually reasonably common issues for plenty of women post-pregnancy without having suffered from HG. However, for those of you who vomited hundreds, if not thousands, of times during pregnancy, incontinence and piles may be an ongoing issue long after the pregnancy is over.

As if peeing when you vomited wasn't awful enough whilst pregnant, discovering that you continue to keep the manufacturers of incontinence pads in business once baby is born and the vomiting has ended could be the final straw! If you find that it is an ongoing issue post-pregnancy, please do bring it up with your midwife or your GP at your 6 week check. They will be able to assess your symptoms and work with you to deal with them. Pelvic floor exercises are key to improving continence, and this is an aspect you can pro-actively help yourself with. Have a look online for how to do effective pelvic floor exercises. There are links on the Spewing Mummy website and NHS Choices also provides up to date information about doing pelvic floor exercises.

The same goes for haemorrhoids (piles). Most women expect some haemorrhoids, especially after giving birth. They are as common a pregnancy symptom as 'morning sickness', although far less talked about. They should shrink on their own after pregnancy but if they continue to be an issue or are particularly troublesome, then do talk to your GP about them. If you suffered from constipation during pregnancy either due to an inability to eat and drink a decent amount or thanks to the side effects of certain medications such as ondansetron, then you may have suffered from piles long before labour and birth. But if they continue to be an issue post-pregnancy or you are having any other bowel-related issues (such as a continuation of constipation), then your GP or practice nurse are the best people to talk to.

Don't suffer in silence – you'll have probably felt like you lost your last ounce of dignity during pregnancy and birth anyway, so don't feel like this is something you should be embarrassed to discuss with anyone. Your GP will have heard it all many times before and will want to try and help you deal with the issue. Many practice nurses have specific skills in continence and bowel management and you may find them a bit more approachable if you are nervous or feeling embarrassed.

Muscle Weakness and General Fitness Levels

Although it may feel truly miraculous to be able to walk around, eat, drink, and generally do everything a 'normal' person does once the pregnancy is over and you are no longer sick (or carrying around an ever-increasing bump!), you may still find that your general fitness level is pretty low and your body finds everyday activities far more exhausting than they should be.

To be fair, many new mums take a little time to regain their usual strength and stamina, as pregnancy takes a fair bit out of even those who sail through pregnancy without any problems. And let's not forget that giving birth is a bit like running a marathon, then there are the sleepless nights of those newborn days which are enough to exhaust anybody. But for somebody who has just survived 9 months of severe sickness, the effects can be much more pronounced.

Let's start with the many, many weeks and months when you were unable to eat anything beyond a few 'safe' foods (if that) and let's add in the many hours spent lying in bed hoping to avoid another bout of vomiting and actually keep some of that food inside your stomach. That in itself is bound to zap your strength and make you a little out of practice when it comes to anything from walking up and down the stairs several times a day, chasing older children as they play, right through to walking into town for a little fresh air and a change of scenery. These may all have been things you dreamed of doing during pregnancy, and whilst it can feel so wonderful to be able to do them, do not be alarmed if they exhaust you more than they used to.

It will take you some time to build up your strength again and get used to these activities, but you will get there. You wouldn't try running a 10-mile race without first building up your strength and stamina, but gradually, you would get there and be able to complete the race. So don't feel too deflated if even the smallest things exhaust you in the early days – take it slowly and gradually do more each day.

However, whilst this is all understandable, please remember that, as with everything else, if you are worried about any of this, then do discuss it with your GP.

Dental Problems

For many women, dental problems are an inevitable consequence of hyperemesis as the acidic vomit damages the enamel and brushing your teeth seems impossible for months on end. There is information in chapter 6 about how to reduce the impact of hyperemesis on your teeth although some women won't be able to do any of those things.

As soon as you have recovered from the birth and are able to get out of the house, make an appointment with your dentist for a thorough check-up and advice about how to help your teeth recover from the trauma. Deal with any new problems as promptly as you can.

Nausea, Panic Attacks, and Other Reactions to Triggers and Flashbacks

We will cover the mental health legacy of HG in the following chapter as it deserves a chapter of its very own. However, it is important to cover the occasional flashbacks which many women experience in this chapter as well, because whilst they may coincide with postnatal depression and PTSD, they are not limited to those affected by these and can affect anyone at any time.

In fact, flashbacks can and do occur at the most unexpected moments and could happen months, even years, after your pregnancy without any warning. They can range from a mild sensation of nausea brought on by the memory of something right through to a full-blown panic attack as you feel yourself transported back to the worst days of your HG hell.

Flashbacks usually have a trigger, and whilst some of these can seem obvious, others may be less so. It could be a certain time of year that reminds you of the months you spent in bed sick, the memory of which fills you with a certain sense of dread and anxiety. It might be a particular song that was popular during your worst days or the theme tune to a television programme your older children used to watch as you tried to rest – these sounds are regularly mentioned as causing a feeling of nausea if ever heard post-pregnancy. It could even be a certain hand soap, washing detergent, or deodorant that was used during your pregnancy and you had forgotten about until the moment you come across it again and find yourself rushing to the toilet trying not to lose your lunch. Smells can be particularly evocative for triggering memories.

Whatever the cause, it must be stated clearly here that the reaction to these triggers is a very physical and distressing one. You may well find yourself banning the use of certain products in your house or asking people not to play a certain tune whilst you are in earshot in an attempt to avoid experiencing a repeat of such an unpleasant reminder. And as with many aspects of HG, you may find people unsympathetic to the severity of your reaction to these triggers; they may even question the validity of it all. Which is why it is important for us to note this as a common experience and so if you experience this, you will know you are not alone.

Damaged Friendships

We couldn't end this chapter without a short note about the damage that a HG pregnancy can do to many seemingly strong friendships. The authors have each experienced difficult relationships due to their own pregnancies and have come across similar stories from almost every woman who has ever had HG. So whilst it can be heartbreaking to lose friends and fall out with family over the way you were supported (or not, as the case may be) during your pregnancy, we felt it crucial to share that again, you are never alone in this experience.

Suffering from any kind of health issue can put a huge amount of strain on any relationship, but when the condition you are experiencing is both misunderstood and unexpected, it can cause far more pain than another condition where the symptoms are both widely known and accepted as part and parcel of the condition. By this, we mean that most people expect pregnancy to be a wonderful and exciting time in your life and so they can find it incredibly difficult to grasp that it can be the most traumatic and terrifying time in your life, especially if they do not see you at your worst because you feel too sick to have any visitors.

Some friendships may be repaired through honest conversations and the desire on both parts to overcome the misunderstanding. After all, sometimes people say truly hurtful things without ever meaning them to be that way, and given the chance to understand what you are going through or have already been through, they will realise how hurtful their comments were and work with you to rebuild the trust and friendship you enjoyed prior to your HG experience.

However, others may seem impossible to save, and this is the most difficult when the relationship is with someone within the family or a friendship group where you have no choice but to make amends because you need to, even if you do not feel you'll ever regain that friendship again. It can be these relationships where the phrases, 'See, wasn't it all worth it in the end?' and 'So when will you be having another?' crop up time and again. Despite your attempts to express how traumatic your experience was, they just do not seem to listen.

Unfortunately, there isn't much you can do about those who do not want to know and you have to make the decision that is right for you and your family. Those friends who want to be there for you will take on board what you say, the others – well, you have to make a decision about whether they are worth fighting for or best ignored.

Either way, we know that these damaged relationships can have a huge impact on your emotional and mental well-being; in fact, they can have as big an impact as the physical symptoms themselves, and so we hope that the following chapter and the contacts at the end of this book may help you to deal with these if you are having problems with friends and family.

Sex and Intimacy after HG

It is natural for sex and intimacy with your partner to go through periods of different activity level, times of drought and times of abundance. Sex certainly isn't the be all and end all of relationships and it's important to keep it in perspective, but it is important nonetheless. Or rather intimacy is important. A relationship without intimacy is far more likely to start deteriorating and have problems than one in which an active life in the bedroom is regularly enjoyed as a couple.

It's not uncommon for a couple's sex-life to decline somewhat after normal pregnancy and birth for a whole host of reasons such as exhaustion from sleepless nights, problems with scar tissue around your labia or vagina causing discomfort and lack of confidence in your post-partum body.

However, for women who have suffered hyperemesis there can be additional issues which reduce enjoyment in sex and intimacy within an otherwise happy relationship. Fear of pregnancy and lack of confidence in contraception is totally understandable after a pregnancy which nearly killed you. However, fears and anxiety need to be dealt with, got in perspective and brought under control... otherwise they control you and can ruin your life (and that of your partner).

> *That's the fear for me, not another child but the being sick and remembering being so sick and just wanting it to stop. Sex suddenly isn't as fun, relaxing and carefree any more cos YOU COULD GET PREGNANT!*

(Anon – HG Survivor)

Other issues that women have reported include feeling like a failure due to the pregnancy, feeling un-feminine and feeling like a disappointment to their partner. And it's not always the women who are fearful of pregnancy and therefore nervous or anxious about sex, our men folk can be just as traumatised by hyperemesis gravidarum and scared that if their partner got pregnant again they would not be able to cope or that she might even die from it. They need as much support and understanding as if it were the other way around.

So lets address how to start dealing with the issues. First of all, ***talk to your partner!*** Get the kids to bed, open a bottle of wine, turn the TV off and talk. Don't book a babysitter and go out for a date-night to talk as you're likely to feel very self conscious in a restaurant or pub and the conversation may get emotional, so stay at home. Tell your partner what's worrying you and how you feel about it. Be as honest and open as you can. Talk about your disappointments over the pregnancy and how it's made you feel in respect to your gender identity and feelings of inadequacy. If it would help then write down key points beforehand. You may find that your partner shares your worries about another pregnancy and be able to offer support and understanding about your other feelings. Or you may find he has been fostering feelings of being inadequate or unattractive to you, which you will also be able to support him in.

Next, *make a plan together!* It is no good to have the conversation and then do nothing proactive to help remedy the issues. A plan needs to be a team effort and should incorporate both of your needs within your comfort zones. There are lots of ways to be intimate which won't result in pregnancy. Mutual masturbation, oral sex and plenty more which will make you feel closer as a couple and help you regain the closeness needed to go on to enjoy penetrative sex. And remember, sex is mean to be a fun, enjoyable experience!

Your plan might include:

- Going together to the doctor or practice nurse to discuss contraception you can both feel confident in. Finding the right contraception for you as a couple may involve compromise and an in depth look at the options.
- Agreeing to turn the TV off every other night for two weeks (for example) and going to bed early to work on your sex life.
- Kissing and cuddling more often.
- Talking about sex openly with each other and talking about the anxiety and fears remaining from the pregnancy.

You could start with agreeing you won't have penetrative sex for a few weeks but focusing on pleasuring each other in lots of other ways. You could also look to build confidence in your body if you have issues around that – your partner clearly taking pleasure in your body is a pretty big boost generally and your partner could agree to help with building your confidence. Women's bodies post baby are never the same as pre-baby but they aren't meant to be and mature men are naturally attracted to their partners' bodies post-baby... you grew his offspring in there!

Maybe talk about fantasies and reminisce on pre-baby antics from your relationship's early days. Play games, dress up, bath or shower together, get outside, wake each other up, but above all, try to have fun and relax.

The purpose of all these suggestions is to build confidence and intimacy but ultimately if you are still very anxious about sex then book to see a counsellor either on your own or as a couple (a link for Relate is in the appendix). Ultimately, if you are careful with contraception so you can't get pregnant then your fears may be bordering on irrational and becoming a phobia... that needs addressing promptly so it doesn't get out of control. If that is the case then please ***get help***.

It's bad enough that hyperemesis gravidarum ruined your pregnancy and perhaps limited your family. Don't let it ruin your relationship or any more of your life.

My youngest is 41 months. We have had sex 6 times since his birth and have not made love for 9 months. I am petrified of getting pregnant and the fear is ruining my life. It is ruining our life.

(Anon – HG Survivor)

There was a deep seated fear of getting pregnant that initially I didn't connect with HG. It took a good few years to figure out that what I was feeling was not an aversion to sex itself, or to my partner but that my body was trying to protect itself from going through another pregnancy. I would experience high levels of anxiety when being physically intimate. It was very confusing and damaging to my self-esteem and my relationship. It was a strong physical response that made me feel out of control of my body. Looked at logically it is completely counter-intuitive to do something (sex) that will result in such a traumatic time, so now I understand it with my brain but my body was still freaking out at having unprotected sex. I would definitely say that HG can cause a level of trauma that significantly affects your experience of intimacy and sex. If it happens to you, you are certainly not alone. Knowing that after my first pregnancy would have been very helpful.

(Anon, HG Survivor)

CHAPTER 11

The Mental Health Legacy of Hyperemesis Gravidarum

During the 1930s in the era of psychodynamic theory development, an opinion was presented that women with HG were mentally ill and that the excessive, life-threatening vomiting was down to a subconscious rejection of the foetus. During the same period the death rate from HG dropped due to the development of intravenous fluid therapy and other anti-emetic treatments. The result of fewer women actually dying, combined with fashionable theories about women's mental states led to abominable treatments where women were literally locked up in mental institutions, prevented from seeing family members, and left in their own vomit for long periods. They even had vomit receptacles removed so they had nowhere to vomit and nurses told not to help them clean up.

Thankfully, on the whole, these sort of stories are rare now, although not entirely unheard of and thanks to staff shortages it isn't uncommon for women in hospital to have to dispose of their own vomit bowls.

Psychological causes for HG have been utterly disproved in more recent years and the psychological impact of HG is beginning to be appreciated, slowly but surely.

There can be no denying that HG can cause mental health issues for the sufferer. And this should really be no surprise when you look at the common experiences of women with HG: the prolonged suffering of continuous, unrelenting nausea and vomiting, vomiting which in itself can be violent, painful, and unpredictable; the isolation of literally months in bed with only minutes a day of company from your partner who is at work the rest of the time, or caring for other children; being unable to read, speak on the phone, watch TV, or gain any respite from focusing on the crippling nausea; the humiliation that comes when vomiting results in urinating on the floor or in your bed or the knowledge you haven't showered in weeks. The list goes on, and quite frankly, it's hardly any wonder depression, anxiety, PTSD, and phobias can ensue.

As there are so many ways in which your mental health may be affected by your experience of HG, we shall look at each one by one.

Perinatal and Postnatal Depression

Perinatal depression describes depression experienced during pregnancy, and postnatal depression is that experienced post birth. Whilst the vast majority of people are aware of postnatal depression, far fewer people are aware of perinatal depression and may even overlook the signs if they are not expecting them.

However, perinatal depression is not uncommon: many women report feeling depressed during pregnancy as a direct result of HG and acknowledging that this is a completely understandable reaction to all you are going through can help you approach your GP or midwife for help in dealing with the depression. A referral to your local perinatal mental health team can make a huge difference in how you cope with the way you're feeling, and they will be able to advise and support you through what is a difficult period.

Getting help is so important because for many women, perinatal depression leads to postnatal depression and that can be far more serious than many people realise – ultimately, for some, it can be fatal. Postnatal depression can lead to all sorts of challenges including difficulties bonding with your baby, resentment of all you have been through and can affect the relationship you have with your partner and other family members, including older children. Postnatal depression can affect anyone, including those who did not suffer from perinatal depression, and so it is important to be aware of the signs to look out for.

Depression is often described as a black cloud that just does not lift, no matter what. It doesn't matter if you feel you should be overjoyed to be pregnant or finally have your new baby home with you, depression eats away at you and colours everything you feel and do. Pretty much everyone expects to feel a little 'blue' and struggle with some things in those early days, but if you find that you are feeling down, anxious, or depressed more than you feel happy and relaxed, then do speak to your GP, midwife, or health visitor about it.

However, please be reassured that this is not the case for everyone. Many women also report feelings of euphoria and wellness like never before after recovering from hyperemesis. Many women also say that nothing seems so hard again and the postnatal phase with a new baby is a walk in the park in comparison to the pregnancy. So please don't assume you will suffer traumatic symptoms after your pregnancy. However, being aware that it is a possibility means that you are better equipped to recognise it earlier and get help quicker.

Postnatal Anxiety

Closely linked to postnatal depression, but worth mentioning in its own right, is postnatal anxiety. Some women find that whilst their mood is generally okay and they are not suffering from post-natal depression they still have a heightened level of anxiety that is affecting their life. Others may find that anxiety goes hand-in-hand with their experience of post-natal depression or PTSD (which will we cover later in this chapter).

A certain amount of anxiety is normal and expected, especially post-pregnancy when you are learning to look after a newborn baby. There is a huge amount of pressure on you to care for this child who relies on you for everything, and it is understandable to worry about whether you are doing everything 'right'. However, anxiety becomes abnormal when it is severe, lasts for long periods of time, or doesn't seem to have a specific cause.

If the anxiety leaves you feeling out of control and as if something awful is going to happen, then it is time to talk to your GP or health visitor about it.

Post-traumatic Stress Disorder

PTSD can be common after a hyperemesis pregnancy. It's hardly surprising if you look at one of the potential causes of the condition – prolonged exposure to an extremely stressful situation. Well, lying in bed for weeks or months on end, vomiting with every movement, and thinking you are dying is pretty stressful. Add in unsympathetic healthcare practitioners, judgemental comments from friends and family, pressure from your workplace, and admission to hospital, and it's clear to see how this can all add up and lead to PTSD.

It is quite common for anyone who has suffered from HG to have the occasional moment of panic or flashback (as mentioned in the previous chapter). It is also relatively common to develop aversions or phobias to certain things (see below) following a HG pregnancy. However for many these will be fleeting moments and occur less frequently as time goes on.

For women with PTSD, this is not the case. The flashbacks can be intense and regular, causing them to 're-live' the experience very vividly and can induce physical sensations such as nausea and vomiting. They can have constant negative thoughts, questioning why it happened and whether they could have done anything differently which can, in turn, lead to feelings of immense guilt or shame. PTSD can also lead women to try and avoid triggers, such as avoiding certain people or places or even avoid the emotions themselves by trying to push the memory out of their minds.

PTSD can spiral rapidly and be terminal so should never be underestimated. If you think that you are suffering from it, then please do contact your GP as soon as possible to access help and support.

Phobias and Aversions

Following a hyperemesis pregnancy, you may find that you have aversions to certain things, particularly certain foods and smells which were triggers for vomiting. You may find that you simply do not fancy these things again after they made you sick, or you may find that the taste, smell, or even just hearing their name or seeing their label can turn your stomach. These aversions may diminish over time, or you may find that you never really enjoy something you previously liked just because of the connection they now have to an awful time in your life. However, these aversions are usually relatively small and easy to avoid and therefore do not have a major impact on your life post-HG.

Phobias, however, can be much more troublesome and may require support through something like cognitive behaviour therapy (CBT) to stop them taking over your life. Phobias are an irrational fear of something and can include emetophobia (fear of feeling and being sick), needle phobia, and an intense fear of hospitals. Whilst these fears may seem completely understandable when you consider that vomiting for months on end, having multiple admissions to hospital, and enduring many attempts to hook you up to an IV for fluids would put anyone off going through it all again, when these fears grow out of control they become a phobia.

Let's look at this another way – nobody likes vomiting, but most people deal with feeling and/or being sick as and when it happens and never give another thought to it. They may feel panicky and hope not to vomit when actually feeling sick; that's a pretty normal response, but they don't worry about it excessively the rest of the time. Someone with emetophobia, however, may try to avoid the possibility of getting sick even when there is no real threat of exposure to anything that could make them vomit anyway. This could include avoiding eating out, drinking alcohol, or visiting friends whose kids have been sick several days earlier, etc. It is the fear of the potential for something to make you sick which is the problem, because it is this which affects the way you live.

Equally, if you find yourself avoiding going to see your GP when you are ill for fear that they may prescribe medications you cannot cope with, order blood tests, or refer you to the hospital, then this fear is out of hand and needs to be addressed.

Treatment and Support Options for Mental Health Issues

You may suffer from one or all of the above conditions, but luckily, they are all treatable, and the first thing you must do if you think you are suffering is to admit that you need help. Then get help! Don't just ignore it and hope you'll get better. When you are suffering from a mental health condition, you need help and support to get through it, even though this may be the last thing you feel able to ask for.

If you are reading this and think a loved one is suffering, then you need to seek help for them, because they may be unable to ask for it themselves. Talk to them and express your concerns, but if you are met with resistance and denial, then don't be put off getting help for them. You may want to wait until they are able to ask for the support themselves, but that may be a long time coming, and in the meantime, their condition could get much worse.

Treatment options vary depending on a wide variety of considerations such as what the issue is, how severe it is, and how you feel about the treatment options offered to you. You may be offered medications to help deal with feelings of depression or anxiety. You may be offered a referral to your local mental health team for counselling, Cognitive Behaviour Therapy, and ongoing support. If symptoms are severe, you may be given the contact details for the crisis team, who can respond to you immediately at any time.

In Appendix 1, we have included contacts for organisations that may be able to help. If your GP or midwife were helpful, then you could try them for a referral to a local service. Postnatal depression tends to be well recognised and supported these days, and you will hopefully be met with empathy and kindness if you seek help for this. Unfortunately though, peri-natal depression and HG-related PTSD tend to be a little less recognised, and it may be harder to get a diagnosis for these. Things are slowly improving, but if your first attempt to get help fails, then try, try, and try again using the avenues listed in the appendix.

Ask your partner to help explain things, and show him the section on advocacy in chapter 7, which can be applied to advocating about anything really, including advocating on your behalf when discussing mental health conditions. But above all, get help. It's bad enough that you suffered in pregnancy – don't let the legacy of HG ruin any more of your life – take control and get help!

Finally, we'll say it again – don't suffer in silence – get help!

CHAPTER 12

Trying again - Preparing for an HG Pregnancy

Despite the old adage that every pregnancy is different, when it comes to HG pregnancies, that's unfortunately not true. If you have suffered once, you have around an 86% chance of suffering again in the next pregnancy to an equal, lesser, or greater degree. On the plus side that leaves a 14% chance of not suffering again and this does on occasion happen.

Although there is no harm in hoping for the best, it is always sensible to prepare for the worst; if you don't need the plans you have in place, then no more harm is done than a little wasted time. Making the decision to have another HG pregnancy can be a big deal for women and their partners, especially if you now have a child to care for whilst ill. If you have decided that you are ready and able to try for another baby, then there are several things you can do in advance to prepare yourself and your family in case HG occurs again.

If you are trying again after a termination or miscarriage, then don't rush yourself. Take time to grieve and heal.

Planning and preparation is unlikely to avoid the occurrence of HG, but it can make coping with and surviving another pregnancy more achievable and may reduce the overall severity of symptoms. One of the major difficulties for women facing hyperemesis for the first time is the sudden onset of symptoms and lack of knowledge and support. That's where you have a head start this time.

By preparing yourself and your family and friends before the pregnancy begins, you can somewhat limit the stress by having coping strategies and support networks in place. A hyperemesis pregnancy will never be easy, but it certainly could be easier.

The following suggestions are just that – suggestions, based on research papers and the experiences of a variety of women who have been through more than one pregnancy. I wish we could say, 'Do all of these things and you'll be okay,' but that's not realistic. What you can do will depend on your personal circumstances, and your plan needs to be workable in your life.

There are two aspects to planning for an HG pregnancy. The first is to do with pre-emptive treatment and having a care plan in place with your health-care providers. The second is to do with lifestyle preparation and support.

Pre-emptive Treatment and Putting a Plan in Place

Experiences differ but one of the most commonly shared experiences amongst HG sufferers is the difficulty in getting the severity of symptoms recognised and adequate treatment offered as early as possible.

Yet early treatment may help limit the overall severity of symptoms. Recent research carried out by the Motherisk Program in Canada showed a significant improvement in symptoms when pre-emptive treatment was used for women who had previously had an HG pregnancy. For the study, the researchers recruited 30 women who called their helpline asking advice in planning for another pregnancy after suffering HG or severe NVP symptoms in a previous pregnancy. All of these women were advised to begin taking anti-emetic medication either as soon as they got a positive pregnancy test or, at the very latest, on the first day of the very first symptom of NVP. The severity of their symptoms was followed by the research team, and a 43.3% reduction in symptom severity was seen.

In order to compare these results with a control group, 29 women who called the helpline once already pregnant and experiencing hyperemesis or severe NVP for a second time were advised to begin taking the anti-emetic as soon as possible. In this group of women, a 17.2% reduction in symptom severity was seen.

This study appears to show a significant difference in the improvement rates of symptoms based in whether anti-emetic medication was taken prior to the onset of symptoms or once they had already begun. It seems that the early use of anti-emetic drugs prior to the onset of symptoms may improve the experience of the mother and prevent the escalation of NVP symptoms to full-blown HG.

The study was based on the idea that medications for motion sickness are taken before travel, and those for post-operative and chemotherapy-induced nausea are given prior to the surgery or treatment and therefore the onset of symptoms. The researchers questioned why such a practice isn't used for treating women at high risk of developing HG in a second or subsequent pregnancy.

The study has its limits, such as the small number of women included in each group and the fact that the choice of anti-emetic used was left up to the women's healthcare provider. However, the results are worth considering when planning another pregnancy of your own.

The author, Caitlin Dean, saw success with this strategy in her own third pregnancy and is an advocate for early treatment.

So which medications should you try? More detailed information about the various treatment options is available in section 1 of this book, and information on the PSS website will reflect the most current research and guidelines available. However, with pre-emptive treatment, it is always worth starting on the first rung of the ladder (see below) before rapidly moving on if this is not enough to control symptoms.

Many women who tried 'baseline' medications such as cyclizine or promethazine in a previous pregnancy may have found they were not effective and needed to move on to stronger medications. This may be because treatment wasn't given until her symptoms were already very severe and getting them under control was more difficult. However, as we have seen above, if started early enough, these baseline medications may be all that is required to prevent an escalation of symptoms. And as these baseline medications have the most safety data available, they are always worth trying first.

An appropriate treatment ladder is available at the end of chapter 4 and can be downloaded from the Spewing Mummy website.

So how do you go about getting pre-emptive treatment? Your first port of call is likely to be your GP, so make an appointment to discuss pre-conception planning with her. There is no reason why the plan cannot be made entirely with your GP. If she is reluctant to make a pre-emptive plan or prescribe the appropriate medication, then it is worth asking for a referral to a local consultant who may have more experience in treating hyperemesis and feel more confident prescribing the medications. However, it is still worth having an appointment with your GP to discuss the plan as it is likely you will need to see her once you are pregnant and so knowing she is happy with the plan in advance will give you more confidence approaching her when needed. If your GP is particularly reluctant, then it is a good idea to change surgeries before you get pregnant so that you have a GP you can work with and have confidence in.

Whether the plan is to be made with a consultant or your GP, it is worth doing a bit of preparation in advance of the appointment. The intention of the following questions is to help you think clearly and realistically about what did and didn't work for you in your last pregnancy and what you would like to try this time. It might be a good idea to photocopy these pages to fill out, or alternatively, you can download them from the PSS or Spewing Mummy websites.

Questionnaire prior to planning next pregnancy

Think about your care providers:

Was your GP supportive and sympathetic?	Yes	No
If No, is changing GP an option?	Yes	No
Did you see a consultant and was he/she helpful?	Yes	No
*If your consultant previously was good, then ask to be referred for a pre-pregnancy consultation them	Yes	No
Was your midwife helpful and supportive?	Yes	No
If No, is there the option of other midwives in the area?	Yes	No
Were your family and friends helpful and supportive?	Yes	No
Have you got plans for childcare in place if required?	Yes	No

Your current state of health:

Are you fit and healthy?

Height ....

Weight ....

Use Google to work out your BMI ....

Do you need to put on weight or lose some weight before this pregnancy? It is good to have some reserves to lose, but it is not good to be overweight – write your own plan here:

....

....

....

In your last pregnancy, which medications helped and which didn't:

Last pregnancy I tried: Buccastem, pyridoxine (vitamin B6), promethazine, cyclizine, Stemetil, metoclopramide, ranitidine, Omeprazole, domperidone, ondansetron (alongside lactulose), steroids,

other..
(delete/add as a appropriate)

Other things I tried: Hypnotherapy, acupuncture and acupressure bands, ginger capsules (250 mg × 4 per day),

other..

What worked ....

What did not work...

Side effects I experienced...

I do not want to try... again.

The most helpful medications were ....

....

....

Medications I did not try last time but would like to discuss with the doctor this time are...

....

Were you able to keep oral medications down?	Yes	No	
Were you offered soluble medications or suppositories?	Yes	No	
Was acid reflux a problem?	Yes	No	Not sure
If Yes, were you given treatment for it?			Not sure

Hospital admission:

If you were admitted to hospital during your last pregnancy, how did you find it? ....

For example, a relief to be in hospital and receiving fluid and medication IV or distressing and stressful ....

....

....

....

If you found it stressful and distressing, can you pinpoint why? For example, admission via A&E, unsympathetic staff, disturbed sleep, busy ward, smells, sensory stimulation, separation from husband/children, etc., side effects from treatments, needle phobia.

....

....

....

If you had the option of IV fluids as a day patient, did you prefer that?	Yes	No

Do you know about other services in your local area, such as Hospital at Home or Acute Care at Home as an alternative to hospital admission?

....

Preparing for your next pregnancy:

Do you hope to try pre-emptive medication?	Yes	No

Other medications I wish to be considered: Buccastem, pyridoxine (vitamin B6), promethazine, cyclizine, Stemetil, metoclopramide, ranitidine, Omeprazole, domperidone, ondansetron (alongside lactulose), steroids, other...
(delete/add as a appropriate)

Hospital admission:

- Do you want to request day patient treatment if it is available? Bear in mind there are pros and cons, such as extra travelling and extra needles for new IV sites!
- If you went through A&E last time, can you avoid that this time?

- Do you have a preferred hospital to go to?

Once you have answered all these questions for yourself, you will hopefully feel more able to discuss a potential plan with your doctor. So, for example, if your consultant suggests you try ondansetron but last time you had it and the constipation was so awful, you had to stop taking it, tell him that, and ask if you could have a laxative prescribed alongside it, such as lactulose.

Now you have thought about what you do and don't want to try in your next pregnancy and you have your appointment lined up, what is the best way to approach your doctor? Go in with a good attitude. Don't assume that the doctor will be dismissive, and don't assume that you will have to 'fight' for treatment. If you are reasonable, then they will have a hard time explaining why they are being unreasonable. That said, unfortunately, it's not always that easy and you may well be met with, 'Oh, every pregnancy is different. Let's wait and see if you get sick.' If that's what you get, you either need to persevere and try to explain why you would prefer to 'plan for the worst and hope for the best' or you need to find a different doctor.

Here are some tips for approaching the consultation:

- Start by explaining that deciding to have another pregnancy has been a difficult decision due to how ill you were last time but that you would desperately like to have another baby and would like their support to get through it.

- Explain why you would like to plan in advance, that is, you have read lots of research and understand that the chances of having it again are very high but that the severity can be reduced by starting treatment early.

- Explain that once you are pregnant and sick, you find it very hard to advocate for yourself as even talking is difficult, so by having an agreed treatment plan in advance, both you and your doctor will know you are comfortable with the drugs being used and your partner will feel more confidence in caring for you at home.

- Make it clear you would like to take responsibility for your condition and work in partnership with them to manage it as best you can.

It helps if you can try to appreciate that many GPs find HG a particularly difficult condition to treat, and many have been trained to be reluctant to prescribe in pregnancy. When a medication is prescribed off-license, as all anti-emetics in the United Kingdom are during pregnancy, it is the responsibility of the prescribing doctor and his professional registration.

The following care plan may be useful for you to fill out in advance as an example of the treatment schedule you would like to use for your pregnancy. Points can then be either agreed to by your doctor or they can explain why it is not appropriate for your case. You can photocopy these pages, or you can download the full care plan from the PSS website.

Pre-pregnancy Care Plan

Before pregnancy/while trying to conceive, I will take:

Treatment	**Tick by patient**	**Tick by GP/script given**
Folic acid		
B6/pyridoxine (10 mg 3 or 4 × a day)		
Other		

Once I am pregnant, I want to start taking:

Treatment	**Tick by patient**	**Tick by GP/script given**
Cyclizine (50 mg 3 × a day)		
OR Promethazine (Avomine) (25 mg 3 × a day)		
And (continue with) B6/pyridoxine (10 mg 3 or 4 × a day)		
Other		

If my condition still worsens, the following criteria will indicate needing to move on:

Treatment	**Preferred route of administration, (delete as appropriate):**	**Order of preference to try**	**Tick by doctor and dose/route to prescribe:**
Prochlorperazine (Stemetil)	Oral/IM injection		
Metoclopramide (Maxolon)	Oral/IM injection		
Ondansetron (Zofran)	Oral tablets/ oral melts/ suppositories/ injection		
Domperidone (Motilium)	Oral		
Other			
Other			

In addition to anti-emetic medication, I would also like to have an antacid treatment, particularly if my symptoms continue beyond the first trimester.

I would like to try omeprazole/ranitidine (delete as appropriate).

Notes:

....

....

....

....

....

Indications for requiring IV Fluids/admission to hospital:

Symptom	**Indication to move on, tick:**	**Method of monitoring (delete as required):**	**Agreed by doctor:**
Vomiting preventing intake of oral medication/not responding to medication		Patient reporting	
Ketones in urine		Patient reporting (Ketostix required)/ urine tested by surgery	
Weight loss >10% of pre-preg weight		Patient reporting/ weighing at surgery	
Fluid intake <500 ml per day, despite medication		Patient reporting	
Urine output <500 ml per day despite medication or not passing urine for more than 12 hours		Patient reporting	
Other			
Other			

Notes:

....

....

....

....

....

Indications for requiring IV Fluids/admission to hospital:

Service	**Available in area?**	**Preferred option (write preference 1st, 2nd, etc)**	**Doctor's comments/ referral to be arranged.**
IV hydration at home via local Acute Care Service	Yes/No		
IV hydration as day patient at ....hospital	Yes/No		
Admission to ....hospital	Direct referral to ward available Yes/No		
Other			

Notes:

....

....

....

....

....

Another matter to discuss at this point with your GP or consultant is your preferred methods of communication. Many doctors like to use email these days, and for the hyperemetic woman, this can be ideal as smart phones enable you to use email from your sickbed as easily as texting and is often preferable to speaking on the phone. If this isn't an option, find out the contact details for their secretary or the best times to call the surgery for getting hold of your GP.

You should also note with your consultant/GP who they may discuss your condition and treatment with them if you are unable to do so yourself. One of the authors, Caitlin, found during her second pregnancy that a GP wouldn't speak to her husband even though she was too sick to speak herself. You could give permission for anyone to speak on your behalf, not just your husband. Perhaps you want your mother, sister, mother-in-law, or even a nanny or au pair to be able to speak to your GP if there are times when they will be the only other adult in the house. It is also worth having their names documented at the GP surgery for attending with any other children you have if they are due immunisations or treatments during your pregnancy. Fathers don't need extra permission on record but nannies, grandparents, aunts, and uncles all will, and it saves an extra hassle during pregnancy if it is recorded in advance.

In some areas, you may be able to get a midwife allocated earlier, and they may be happy to act as a point of contact between yourself and the GP or consultant. Whoever is involved in your care though should get a copy of the care plan. It can be scanned onto your electronic notes at the GP surgery, and you should keep a copy yourself.

All of this may sound daunting, but having a plan in place that your consultant and GP have agreed to follow will hopefully reduce the need for fighting for acknowledgement and medication once you are pregnant. It will be easier to discuss this with a clearer mind prior to pregnancy than once the symptoms begin to kick in, especially considering how quickly the symptoms can escalate for some women. It will hopefully also help you and your partner to feel empowered to get through the tough times ahead, knowing that at the very least you won't have a battle on your hands with your healthcare providers. The only thing you have to battle now is the HG itself.

Lifestyle Preparation and Support

Personal Preparation

Once you have your pre-emptive treatment plan in place, you may want to look at the lifestyle changes and plans you can put in place to help when you are pregnant. On a personal level, there are a number of steps you can take to get yourself 'HG fit'. For example, while you may be tempted to put on a little extra weight in order to have reserves to lose, we don't advocate that as a good idea. It is better to go into pregnancy from a healthy starting weight and as fit as you can be. The exception is if you are currently underweight, in which case it is a good idea to try to get your weight up to a healthier weight if you can. A healthy and normal BMI (body mass index) range is 18.5 to 24.9 so for a woman planning an HG pregnancy we would suggest aiming for the upper end of that, say 23 to 24.9 being ideal (use an online chart or calculator to work out your own BMI, a link is available on the Spewing Mummy website).

Start eating little and often now. If you normally have two slices of toast for breakfast, then start having one slice at normal time and then the other slice an hour or so later. Eating little and often is one self-help technique that really does work for a lot of women. It doesn't help for everyone, and women who can't keep any food or fluid down are unlikely to be helped by force feeding themselves only to increase the emesis. Before your symptoms get very severe though, eating little and often can help enough to prevent significant deterioration, and the earlier you start changing your eating habits, the easier it will be to continue when you are feeling nauseated and horrid.

Add protein to every snack. Some nuts, cheese, or meat should be a major proportion of everything you eat. For more information on dietary tips, see the chapter on self-help.

See your dentist for a check up: although it's free once you're pregnant you are very unlikely to go once you're sick. Get any outstanding issues, such as fillings, resolved and really look after your teeth as best you can before pregnancy so they will cope better during the months you struggle with brushing.

Preparing Your Household and Finances

Household preparation will depend very much on your personal circumstances. Sit down with your partner and write down all of the details you need to sort out and then mark them off as and when you have them sorted.

Let's address employment first. If you work, can you talk to your employer in advance, explaining the situation and discussing the possibility for flexible working, working from home, or perhaps a leave of absence? Depending on your work and your level of illness, these may or may not be options, but knowing where you stand and checking what benefits and sick pay you are entitled to before you fall pregnant could save a lot of stress later on. You may want to speak to your union representative or request to see occupational health for more information and guidance. Citizens' Advice or Maternity Action may also be able to advise you on your rights as an employee, and there is information on the PSS website.

Your partner may also want to discuss the situation with his or her manager as flexible working may make things easier. They could check out what rights they have to compassionate leave if you are suddenly admitted to hospital or there are problems with your childcare arrangements.

If you are able to afford a nanny who will take care of household washing, cleaning, and cooking meals, then great! However, if affording a nanny isn't an option (which it isn't for most families), look at what help you can afford: an au pair, a cleaner for a few hours a week, a childminder, a laundry service which picks up and drops off, or none of those. If the answer is none of those, then what free help is available? Do grandparents live nearby to help with childcare or to help look after you? Are you happy for your mother-in-law to help clean your house or do your washing? Can your partner change their working hours a little to accommodate school/nursery drop off and pickup?

Talking of drop off and pick ups from school or nursery, it may be a good idea to discuss the situation with your child's teacher or nursery staff and provide a list of the people who have permission to pick up your kids. If there might be a number of people, then setting up a password for collecting your child which the staff are all aware of is an effective way of managing this. You could also explain to the staff that your child may struggle emotionally over the coming months if things at home are difficult or mum is in hospital and that they may need extra support with this. There is an excellent children's book available called Mama Has Hyperemesis Gravidarum, But Only for a While by Ashli Foshee McCall, which can help explain what is happening. Perhaps you could provide a copy for their teacher or nursery key worker to read with them. It is an American book and so the treatment options and language used are slightly different to the United Kingdom but is still a great book. I, Caitlin, used this book with my children in my second and third pregnancies and found it really helpful as did many other families I know.

Perhaps you have no family nearby and your partner works long hours in a high-pressured career. How will you cope if you need admitting to hospital? Are there friends nearby to help with childcare or perhaps do some shopping for you? How do you feel about letting your little one watch hours of television and perhaps not even leaving the house for a day? In reality, a few weeks of intensive TV or DVD viewing while you lie on the sofa with a sick bucket is highly unlikely to harm them, but if it bothers you, what other activities might they be able to do with minimal input from you? See the website list in the back for Adventures of Adam which has specific activities for mums suffering HG to maximise child distraction with minimal effort from mum.

Does anyone you know have a teenage son or daughter who would like to earn few pounds taking your little one to the park for an hour or so? Could they go via the shop on the way home and pick up the milk, bread, and baked beans?

Many women in this day and age find it very hard to ask for help from friends. We are expected to cope within our nuclear family units and to get on with things or to pay for help in the form of cleaners and nurseries. But actually, many people are only too happy to have the opportunity to help a friend who is suffering but often don't know how best to help. If you allocated 'godparents' to your child/children, then this is their opportunity to spend quality time with them. Let them take them out for the day while you rest. Ask them to text you pictures through the day so you can enjoy seeing the fun they are having.

Preparing physically and mentally can make the 9 months ahead seem more manageable and help you feel ready to face them head on. Buy yourself a set of plastic mixing bowls – make them your sick bowls. You can ceremoniously chuck them out at the end of pregnancy. Before my third pregnancy, I, Caitlin, bought a set of 3 blue bowls, a big one, a medium one, and a slightly smaller one; they stacked inside each other. They were great because everyone knew they were my sick bowls. When I'd announce, 'Quick, get me a sick bowl,' they were easy to spot. The small one was the one I took around the house with me, and the bigger one stayed by the bed. By having three, one could be emptied (by my devoted husband) while I was filling the next.

Indulge in a new set of pyjamas and slippers that you will feel comfortable in day and night for weeks and weeks. Other treats to prepare yourself might be a new pillow or bedsheets. A new bedside lamp or a television for the bedroom. Basically, anything that is going to make you feel more prepared to cope with what lays ahead and to add touches of comfort to an otherwise miserable pregnancy.

Finally, here are some other tips which may or may not help you in your personal preparations. If you don't yet have any children, then many of these things might not be relevant, but if you have two young children at home, then some of these could be life – or marriage – savers when you are at your worst points:

- Set up online grocery shopping that is delivered to your door. Try to think about the essentials you will need each week and have a 'standard list' saved that you can add to as and when you want to. Most supermarkets enable you to save essential items to a list in your account, and some automatically ask you if you need your 'regular' items. These could include bread, milk, and items for your partner's or child's lunchbox.
- Make lots of ready meals in the freezer for your partner and children and stock up on tins soups, beans, and so on.
- If any of your appliances, such as the washing machine, are not entirely straight forward to use (perhaps the symbols on the dial are worn away), then write out instructions for its use so that your partner, mother, or any one else can use it easily.
- If you have specific requirements, for example, you don't use biological washing powder for the children's clothes, then write it all down. Perhaps in a 'household manual'.
- Make sure you are stocked up on things that your partner may not have a clue about, such as vacuum bags, bathroom cleaning products, and so on. Write in the household manual where all these things are so you don't have to explain the spot, at the back of the cupboard or under the stairs where the spare light bulbs are, while you have your head down the loo – or via text from the hospital.
- If you have a landline then get a cordless one with an answer phone or caller display. You can have it by the bed, sofa, or in the bathroom if you

are waiting for the doctor to call, but you can screen non-essential calls. Remember, if you are screening calls with an answer phone make sure your doctor knows as many will hang up if an answer phone answers.

- Load an MP3 player up with audiobooks, podcasts, and relaxing music.
- If you can afford an e-book reader such as a kindle, then it could be a great investment as they are easy to use in bed lying on one side and turning pages requires minimal movement with one finger. If not (and you think you may be able to read normal books), have a stash of favourite reads, easy reads, or even some new titles by your bed.
- Get some apps on your smart phone, such as solitaire – they engage your mind enough to distract from the nausea but don't take any real effort or movement.
- You may want to get scent-free soap, baby wipes, and so on to reduce triggers.
- A pill dose box can also be really useful if you find it hard to keep track of your medications, particularly if the medications are making you drowsy or a bit confused.
- Prepare vomit vessels and measurable drink containers.
- Have some activities planned for any children at home in case you have days when you are alone with them. And stock up on DVDs that your child will like but won't be too much of a trigger for you. A lot of the older television series are much slower paced and less sensory stimulating than the new ones. Plus you'll probably enjoy watching Bagpuss over and over again more than the Tweenies!

A lot of this will be less relevant if your previous pregnancy ended in miscarriage or termination and you don't already have a child. In these cases, the need for emotional support will be all the more important for both you and your partner.

Support

Whether or not you have children already, emotional support for the long lonely weeks is essential. One of the lessons that I, Caitlin, learned from going through three hyperemesis pregnancies is that the friends you have who have not had HG themselves, no matter how much they want to support you, are unlikely to be able to provide the actual support you need. It is important to have realistic expectations of your friends so that you are not disappointed and end up with feelings of resentment.

That's not to say you can't utilise your friends, but perhaps take time to reflect on their own strengths and think in advance of specific tasks they can support you in. A friend who is a stay at home mum may be able to take your child to play group with her once a week. A friend who enjoys cooking may be able to make some meals for your partner to keep in the freezer. A friend who works but doesn't have children may pick up some magazines for you and drop them over once a week, or perhaps they could forward on amusing emails or interesting articles for you every now and then.

Make an information pack for close friends and family with helpful information such as triggers you find problematic, for example, smelling of cigarette smoke or garlic, talking about food, etc, which they could avoid when visiting might be useful for them. Perhaps explain that last time you felt very isolated and although you want visitors, it would be helpful if they could text first to check that it's a good time to call by. Explain that keeping in touch via text is particularly useful for reducing isolation.

The emotional suffering experienced during a hyperemesis pregnancy is quite a unique experience and one which can generally only be fully understood by other women who have actually suffered themselves. It is for this reason the charity PSS has developed a national peer support network. More details of the support network are in chapter 6, Coping Strategies, but in terms of preparing for another pregnancy, there is no reason why you can't get in touch with the charity and its support network at the early stage of planning so that they have your details ready to match you once you are pregnant. There is also a support forum on their website which has a section specifically for women planning subsequent pregnancies.

A support network could make a massive difference to your experience, and taking the time to build it up before your pregnancy means it is there when you really need it.

If you found yourself getting significantly depressed in your last pregnancy, or if you suffered postnatal depression or PTSD after a previous pregnancy, then getting some counselling for this may be a good idea. Perhaps investigate

CBT to cope with distressing symptoms and anxiety or panic attacks or if you have a needle phobia or fear of hospitals. You can ask for a referral through your GP, but a lot of services now accept self NHS referrals.

We've discussed a lot in this chapter and not all of it will apply to your personal circumstances. Most important of all, however, is to do what you feel you need to do to prepare yourself for another pregnancy. Take what feels right for you and your circumstances and do it. Forget about the rest. You are the one who has to get through the coming months, and only you know what needs preparing to make it as easy as possible. That said, it is far better to over prepare than under prepare and end up winging it!

Here is a checklist for you to summarise all the suggestions in this chapter:

- Complete the worksheet looking at your previous pregnancy and think about what you would like to do differently this time.
- Have an appointment with your GP and/or consultant to make a plan and get pre-emptive prescription.
- With you partner, make a list of all the matters which will need addressing while you are out of action.
- Create a list of the people who can support you and what they can each do.
- Discuss your plan with family/friends.
- Create an information pack for family/friends.
- Create a household management pack for main carers.
- Go to the dentist for a check-up/clean.
- Contact PSS, register for support, and join the forum to get support there too. Also encourage your partner to get support in the partners' forum.
- Talk to your current children about the pregnancy and how it might affect you all.
- Talk to your manager about flexible working/rights, etc.
- Talk to your children's teacher/key nursery worker/childminder etc about hyperemesis.

- Stock up on food and drinks you tolerated last time.
- Stock up your cupboards and freezer for partner/children.
- Have some activities planned for the children when you are sick.
- Buy essential supplies: Ketostix, wet wipes, mints, sick bowls, sick bags, incontinence pads (weeing while you're sick often starts earlier each pregnancy!), see the Spewing Mummy website for recommended products.
- Make up spare bed if possible/necessary.
- Build up your 'coping station'; snacks, drinks, books or kindle (loaded with books), MP3 player (loaded with audiobooks), DVDs, and anything else to pass the time. Have an easy-to-reach place by the bed or sofa
- Get the Spewing Mummy wall chart for ticking off the days
- Buy cards/presents for birthdays in the year ahead, wrap presents, and write cards so that your partner can just post them at the right time – Amanda's idea, genius!
- Buy or unpack some comfy maternity clothes, particularly pyjamas.
- Buy any baby essentials you will need early on.

CHAPTER 13

Your Family, the Only Child and Adoption

The Only Child

> *After 3 weeks of severe HG, I had a miscarriage. This would have been my second child, a sibling for my 6-year-old. I don't think I can go through it again, so my daughter will have to remain as an only child. I'm heartbroken. I really wanted her to have a brother or sister.*

(Sarah, HG Survivor)

The decision not to have another child due to HG is relatively common. Some women stop at just one child, despite wanting more and others may go on to have a second or third child but feel they have to stop short of the larger family they always dreamed of. Whilst there are a certain number of things you can do to try and make your pregnancy easier, sometimes they just aren't enough and the decision to never face another HG pregnancy is the one that feels right for you.

It is a decision that I, Amanda, made and whilst there were other factors which ultimately added to this decision, the thought of facing hyperemesis again was the biggest factor of all. It wasn't an easy decision, and I spent a good 18 months swinging between thinking I (and my family) could survive another pregnancy and knowing deep down inside that we could never face it again.

The decision led me through a whole range of emotions from fear and heartbreak through to acceptance and even joy in our choice to raise an only child. My husband and I looked at options such as fostering and adoption, and whilst we have still not completely ruled either of those out, we are currently very happy raising our 'one and only'. We feel lucky to have what we have, and it seems we are not alone.

> *I am so lucky just to have one! He will be my one and only because of HG, but hey, what a lucky mummy I am because we survived it! We have so much pressure put on us to have more children but some of us just can't no matter how much we wish we could. I've really struggled with not*

been able to have more children but am just accepting it now and enjoying so very much being a mummy to my one and only amazing boy.

(Sarah, HG Survivor)

One-child families are actually on the rise. Factors such as the rising cost of living and couples choosing to start their families later in life have all influenced the decision many families make regarding how many children they have. But there still seems to be a stigma around choosing to have an only child.

I only want one child – some people treat me as though I'm abnormal!

(Kirsten, HG Survivor)

The idea that only children must be lonely or spoilt still seems to be thrown around in society, and there seems to be a real pressure on women to provide their child with a sibling. Although ironically, women who have more than two children also report feeling pressure to not have any more and a prevailing attitude that they are 'selfish' or 'greedy'.

Despite desperately wanting another baby, both my husband and I are doubtful that I could cope with hyperemesis and the depression it causes. Women in Western society just can't win. You're selfish if you choose not to have children, choose to have one, or choose to have a large family.

(Delphi, HG Survivor)

It seems as if no matter what decision you make regarding your family size, someone will have an opinion about it. But as the most commonly quoted message about only children is that they will be lonely or selfish, we decided it would be helpful to ask someone who grew up as an only child to share his experience and address these concerns.

Mat Connelly, is a friend of the author (Caitlin) and developer of both the PSS and Spewing Mummy websites:

I'm 37, and never once in my life have I wished for a sibling. Being an only child was a truly wonderful experience – I had my parents' undivided attention the whole time! My friends were jealous that I didn't have to share a bedroom with an annoying sibling, wear their hand-me-down clothes, or drag along a younger brother in tow every time we went out to play.

Let me dispel some myths about being an only child:

- *They'll be lonely. I was never short of friends to play with and formed a really close bond with my parents because there wasn't another sibling to compete with for their time. Presumably you're going to let them have friends?*

- *They'll be spoiled. It's true that I got more presents on my birthday than some of my friends with lots of siblings, but that's because my parents weren't so strapped for cash only having one child. Surveys suggest raising a child costs an average of £148,000. Are you sure you want more than one?*

- *They'll be anti-social. To be honest, I find this quite insulting. I've met anti-social only children, yes, but I've also met very anti-social people who have siblings! Bring up your only child in a loving environment, and they'll be well-rounded individuals, just like you.*

- *They'll miss having the kind of relationship that having a sibling provides. I've formed a number of lifelong friendships with people that I consider to be closer than a brother or sister, people to whom I'd donate bone marrow or a kidney without a second thought. I know people who have/had unpleasant, even abusive relationships with their siblings and recent surveys suggest this is more prevalent than people think.*

- *They won't have a brother or sister to help look after me when I'm old. Seriously? If you're just having kids so they can care for you later in life, you're probably so selfish that they won't want to look after you.*

If I've got one regret from my childhood, I wish I'd had a puppy.

The authors would like to express here that we are not saying that having an only child is better or worse than having more than one. It is a completely personal decision that you have to make for yourself, which is highlighted by the fact that the two of us have completely different families: Amanda has an only child, and Caitlin has three children!

However, we do want to make it clear that deciding to have an only child is a perfectly understandable decision to make following a HG pregnancy and that whilst almost everybody will have an opinion on whether or not you should have more children, it is yours and yours alone to make.

My husband and I have decided that we are only having one child. People make comments like, 'Oh, you will soon forget about it all and long for another one.' I won't forget about it easily as it has left me debilitated and I have other complications too. I have been off work for a long time now, so money has been a tight and I have heavily relied on my husband for physical and emotional support. Would I want to put my husband through this again? No! Would I want to be this ill again with a toddler? No! My only child will be very loved as I am just grateful that I can have one child as some can't have any at all. Will he miss out? No! He will have cousins and friends to play with. I won't feel pressurised or be made to feel guilty because of our choice.

(Natalie, HG Survivor)

Adoption – An Alternative to Hyperemesis Gravidarum?

There is no doubt hyperemesis limits an awful lot of families. As discussed above, many women cannot face going through pregnancy again despite wanting more children. Most of them already have one child but sadly some have none.

We have already looked at the decision to raise an only child, and that is indeed the best and most favoured option for some. However, many people do want more than one child, and if going through hyperemesis again is definitely not an option, then an alternative to consider is adoption.

Adoption is an option open to people in the United Kingdom and with over 4,500 children waiting for adoption in the United Kingdom, adoptive parents are desperately needed. However, it is important that people considering adoption because they can't have more children biologically have taken the time to grieve for the babies they haven't had. Counselling may help if you are struggling with this and you should allow yourself to go through the grieving process. Most (though by no means all) of us women have grown up from a young age with ideas about our future family and the children we plan to have so not being able to for whatever reason is a genuine loss and the grief can be profound. Give yourself time to heal and come to terms with it.

The vast majority of local authorities and adoption agencies will not accept your application to adopt until your youngest child is of a certain age, usually around the age of 2 years old, for this very reason. They want to be sure that you have had enough time to come to terms with the idea of never having another child of your own to ensure that you are completely sure you want to adopt. Adoption is an amazing experience for some, but it is important to remember that some adoptions break down and this is why the adoption process is so intense: they want to ensure that both you and the child you adopt are right for each other.

How do you know if adoption is the right choice for you?

Well, to start with, find out as much as you can about adoption. Look online, read blogs about adoption, investigate which agencies there are in your area, and contact your local authority. You'll get invited along to an information meeting where you will find out more about what it means to be an adopter and about the children who need adopting. Here you will meet social workers, experienced adopters, and other people considering adoption. At this point, if you decide to continue, you'll choose an agency to register with.

What happens after you register with an agency?

The process involves two stages.

Stage one involves the background checks, references, and medical/criminal history checks. You also attend workshops to learn more about adoption and the challenges faced when becoming an adoptive parent.

Kate Hilpern, a journalist colleague, has sat on an adoption panel for 10 years and I asked her to explain how adoption differs from standard parenting. Here she explains the challenges and gives a realistic take on the process:

> *Adoptive parenting is often described as therapeutic parenting because it requires an additional set of skills in addition to the usual nurturing and love that being a mother or father requires. Usually, these children come from a damaged past – mainly neglect or abuse – and it's the adoptive parent's job to help the child overcome any challenges that this may have brought them, whether this manifests itself in worrying behaviour, coping with painful memories, dealing with loss or all of those things, and more. If you ask people to imagine the worst case scenario, they'll usually think of a child who is troublesome and wild, but sometimes the opposite problem happens – that is, they are withdrawn, which can be even more difficult to deal with. For most children, it's neither one nor the other but a complex mix of challenges that pop up at different times of their childhood.*

There's no doubt it's challenging, but the vast majority of adoptive parents say it's hugely rewarding and ideally, you should get support when you need it. Having sat on an adoption panel for a decade, it was most satisfying to see these adults who were so keen to be parents either for the first time or to add onto their existing families being matched with children who need homes.

Nobody would say it's easy, and this explains why the adoption process can seem challenging and long. Indeed, with an estimated one in five adoptions breaking down, it's essential that we know for sure that any adults who are approved for adoption are going in with their eyes wide open.

Stage one should only last 2 months although you can take longer over it if you want. If at this point, you still want to proceed, you'll move onto stage two.

This stage is carried out by a social worker and takes around 4 months. The social worker will make a number of visits to your home and you will talk about why you want to adopt and what sort of child would best suit your family. You'll also attend further training sessions which prepare you for becoming adoptive parents.

Next, your case will be presented to a panel which you will be invited to attend. Based on the report and meeting, the panel will give a recommendation and the agency will either approve you or not.

Assuming you get approved, you will then be matched with a child, usually within 3 months, but it can take longer. Often though, it is very quick as agencies explore potential matches before approval in order to speed up the process. But this is not a passive process and you can also proactively look for the right child for you via the family finding service Be My Parent (run by BAAF) and via adoption activity days amongst others.

Once a potential match is found for you, more information about the child or children, including their family background, early years' history, reason for needing adopting, any special needs, and general character will be provided and discussed. If you want to go ahead with the match, then you will attend another panel who will also look at whether it is a suitable match and make a recommendation.

We owe it to these children to make sure a forever family means just that

– not a family who is going to let them down because they were not well prepared enough. Many adults wind up changing their mind about the kind of child they'll take on. Having originally wanted a baby, they might end up preferring the idea of a toddler or an even older child or they might decide to consider a sibling group or a child with disabilities. This also takes time to work through.–

(Kate Hilpern)

Once the match is approved, you get to meet the child. Getting to know them usually starts with a visit to their foster carer's house or planned outings. Next the child will visit you at home, including overnight stays. The child will move in as soon as you are all ready, which will obviously be exciting for you all!

You would be entitled to statutory adoption leave and pay and will continue to be supported by your social worker. Finally, after a minimum of 10 weeks, you can apply to the courts for an adoption order, and once this is complete, the child will be legally yours and can take your surname!

This is a very short overview of what can be a very intensive process. As stated previously, reading blogs of those who have been through the adoption process can be really helpful in getting a clearer idea of what it's like going through the process of adopting a child. There are many UK-based adoption bloggers and a link to some of these are included in Appendix 1 at the back of the book.

We've also asked Fiona and her husband, who adopted a sibling pair, to answer some questions about their experience of becoming adoptive parents to their children:

How did you find the process? *Overall we found the adoption process 'okay' and not too intrusive, as we were warned it might be. Myself and my husband were lucky that we had supportive employers who gave us time off work to have the meetings with our social worker, so this helped. We did feel that some questions weren't particularly relevant, but in the main, understood why we were being asked what we were asked. We found the 4 days training to be extremely worthwhile – they gave us a huge insight into the type of children that are up for adoption and it was also helpful for us to meet other people in a similar situation to us. We were also lucky that we only waited approximately 3 months for a match.*

What fears did you have and were they justified? *Our fears were that the process would be intrusive. This partly came from local authority information events that we went to, which were quite negative. We also thought that the process would be lengthy and time-consuming. Whilst it was quite time-consuming, our social worker was very supportive and encouraging and kept us fully informed of everything throughout the process. It didn't feel as long winded as we thought and we also came to realise that we needed the time to think everything through and feel confident that we were making the right choices.*

Another fear was that all children up for adoption are massively damaged and/or have disabilities and learning difficulties. Whilst the children need support and have obviously had difficult starts, it is not the case that they all are hugely damaged and have special needs.

What has been the best thing about adopting for your family? *The best thing is that we have two fantastic children! We feel that we have 'hit the jackpot' with our children. They are at great ages, and we feel lucky to have missed the baby stages (e.g. sleepless nights and nappies!) They have been fully accepted into the family and ourselves and extended family love and adore them more than words can say.*

What advice would you give to someone considering adoption? *The best piece of advice we were given was to 'shop around' the different adoption agencies. We were very much put off by the local authority info events so decided to go to voluntary agencies and in the end chose one that was a recommendation.*

The other piece of advice would be to 'try and be patient', which is far easier said than done. It's important to carry on with life whilst waiting for a match and make the most of being able to do what you want when you want!

Conclusion

Pressure in society about how families 'should be' is rife, and couples can feel overwhelmed by comments from people about having more children. This can be particularly problematic for women who have suffered hyperemesis as other people cannot understand why 'pregnancy sickness' would prevent them having more. The question about why she is unable to 'put up with just

9 months of sickness for a lifetime of happiness' can come up frustratingly frequently, and it can be an extremely painful and distressing question to answer if you'd actually really love another child but feel unable to do it again.

Although having an only child is perfectly acceptable and women should not be made to feel like they ought to have more or are selfish not to, some couples do want to expand their families. Others may not have any children despite having suffered hyperemesis, sometimes through multiple pregnancies. For these people, adoption may be an option to consider.

It is not the same as having a biological child of your own but that doesn't mean it is not as good – it may even be better! But it does require a thorough process to ensure the child is suitably matched and the adoption will be successful. Time should be taken to grieve for the pregnancies and children which you can't have before exploring adoption.

There are other alternatives such as fostering and surrogacy, but it is beyond the scope of this book to explore all these options.

CHAPTER 14

The Silver Linings – Seeing the Positive in Your Experience

There can be little doubt that HG is a tough experience and it would be great if no one had to suffer it ever. However, until a cause and cure for hyperemesis is found, women will continue to suffer not just the illness but the stigma, cruel comments, and poor treatment that come with it.

If you are reading this book, then chances are your life, or that of someone you love, has been affected by hyperemesis and to find the positives in a miserable situation can only be considered a good thing.

Earlier in the book, we addressed the ongoing physical and mental problems associated with hyperemesis, and whilst we don't want to undermine the ongoing suffering some women experience, we also don't want to paint a picture of doom and gloom. Many women report utter euphoria when they recover from hyperemesis. For most women, it ends the moment the placenta is delivered and can feel like a heavy black cloud is lifted. After that there can be some truly positive things that can come for a person's journey with the condition.

> *I did have hyperemesis. It's part of my story and you know what – I'm glad now... Am I mad? Well, maybe a little but the truth is some really great things have happened because I had HG! And I'm not just talking about my angelic little darlings (ahem). It has been part of my journey and it's made me who I am.*

(Caitlin, HG Survivor, Author)

If you engage in the support available for hyperemesis, you will undoubtedly make friends. Hyperemesis is a truly bonding experience. At the time you may feel totally alone and isolated and find it impossible to believe that anyone else has ever suffered like you are doing, but they have, and are, and will. Connecting with other sufferers is an incredible experience in itself, and to find out you are not the only one who has fantasised about miscarrying a baby you tried for months to conceive and you're not the only one being told to think positively and try ginger, is liberating. By bonding with other women you can gain hope and a strength to survive the condition. United we can make a massive difference not just to our own experience but to thousands of other women too.

I have friends not just around the United Kingdom but around the world, women and their partners whom I am bonded to by hyperemesis gravidarum.

(Caitlin)

Many women list personal growth, compassion, and tolerance as good things that have come out of their battles with hyperemesis.

Most of us like to think we are compassionate people and open-minded to the struggles of others. But in reality, most of us really cannot appreciate the suffering of others and the sheer horror of many people's medical conditions and mental traumas. Hyperemesis sufferers may feel totally alone and misunderstood by HCPs and the world, but we are not alone. There are literally hundreds of misunderstood conditions which are met with equal disbelief, pseudoscience, and old wives' tales. These include various mental health conditions, myalgic encephalomyelitis, fibromyalgia, various allergies, irritable bowel syndrome, SPD to name but a few. At least with HG, it's generally over after 9 months: many other conditions last a lifetime! How many of us would suggest acupressure bands to a chemotherapy patient, homoeopathy to a woman crippled with SPD, or positive thinking for fibromyalgia?

Sadly, hyperemesis sufferers often report losing friends during pregnancy. It can be difficult to cope with feelings of being abandoned by close friends. Understanding that it's simply impossible to understand what HG is like if you haven't been through it may help. It's not through lack of caring, it's a lack of knowing how to care. When you are the ill one, stuck in bed day after day, week after week, it's hard to remember how quickly the weeks fly by when you're at work every day, sorting the kids out, and generally getting on with life – it's a matter of perspective. Tolerating and forgiving your friends' shortcomings are hard skills to master but are positive skills you can get out of hyperemesis. You can decide here and now to be a better friend to others than they have been to you. See tolerance and perspective as things you will gain from this experience and you'll be grateful for it in the long run.

A lot of women report enjoying the newborn phase with their baby all the more for having suffered so badly. After 9 months of constant nausea, there is a physical lightness that comes with being nausea-free.

The pains of labour could be more manageable if you think of each one bringing you closer to wellness and the end of hyperemesis. The sleepless nights aren't nearly so hard when you don't feel sick, and subsequent coughs, colds, and tummy bugs pale in comparison to nine long months of sickness.

On top of that many women report that their relationships and marriages are stronger, thanks to hyperemesis. For the friendships lost, there will be others that have strengthened. A friend who has been there to support and care for you is likely to be considered a true, loyal, and close friend. A partner who has stuck by you, supported and cared for you through the nightmare is likely to make a great Dad and hopefully you will have years of happiness together as a family and a confidence in your relationship that you are a team who tackle problems together.

The Hyperemesis Improvement Movement

Thanks to the proactive approach of the thousands of women involved in the community, there is already significant change happening in the United Kingdom and around the world for hyperemesis sufferers. The aim we should all have is to improve care and treatment for our daughters and nieces so that they don't have to suffer the isolation and battles with doctors we have had to suffer. Even if we can't cure HG for good, we can at least improve the situation for those doomed to suffer it.

Twenty or so years ago women who miscarried in the first trimester were pretty much booted out of the scanning room doors with a 'better luck next time' pat on the head from the doctors and nurses. There was no ongoing support or care. No information or choices about management options. No charity information was provided, and there was very little sympathy. It was considered pretty standard and common, and the feeling of the woman suffering the miscarriage were barely addressed. Now just 20 years on (having suffered two miscarriages myself – Caitlin), the situation could not be more different. Early bleeding is taken seriously and investigated. If a miscarriage is discovered, women are treated with care and compassion. Written information is given about your options for treatment (where applicable) and you are supported to make the choices right for you. You are treated with dignity and given information about charities that can support you. The trauma is acknowledged, and ongoing care into future pregnancies is planned.

That difference, in just 20 years, is what we hope to achieve with hyperemesis care. It is our hope that women are diagnosed quickly, treated with compassion and dignity, given choices, and supported in a way that is right for them. Information about the support available provided as standard and ongoing care provided into subsequent pregnancies. It's an achievable goal and will be made all the more achievable the more women get involved.

We are at the brink right now. The awareness of HG is increasing rapidly. Amazing Green Top guidelines for the United Kingdom will soon be released, and there are more and more blogs and articles being written on the condition. Hospitals are embracing better practice and care for hyperemesis patients, IV fluids are becoming available at home, and the media are taking note of the condition. Healthcare journals are publishing best practice articles, and poor practice is being challenged. We, the mothers of now, can change the situation further for our daughters and nieces and granddaughters. Stand up, take action for your children, your HG Survivors, make them proud, set the example, let them know that they can improve the world, and add compassion and empathy and care to people who are suffering, not just from hyperemesis but all sorts of misunderstood or under-appreciated conditions.

We talk so much of being proud of our children. Well, let's make our children proud of us! Let's make sure that when we tell them about the hyperemesis we suffered during pregnancy, we can add, 'And this is what I did about it... I went on to support other women, I raised money for the charity that supported me, I raised awareness about hyperemesis, I changed practice in my area, I fought for the rights of sufferers, I spoke out about it and advocated for other sufferers'.

So how can you turn your nightmarish experience of hyperemesis into a positive force for change? In the Spewing Mummy Blog that accompanies this book, there are lots of ideas for getting involved in the international hyperemesis community. Coined the 'Hyperemesis Improvement Movement', we hope to really inspire people to take a stand and turn their experience into something really positive for society and individual sufferers.

Raising money for PSS (or the HER Foundation if you are outside the United Kingdom) is a really positive way you can help. There are loads of options from personal challenges to coffee mornings or just regular direct debit donations. See their websites for further ideas about fundraising.

Raising awareness about hyperemesis is also a really positive way to improve care for the masses. If you can write well, then magazines and journals may be interested in your story. Or you could give talks at local parenting groups, midwifery colleges, and medical schools. Lots of GP Surgeries have 'expert patients' for various conditions. Offer to be the expert patient on this condition. Ask if you can put posters and leaflets from PSS in their waiting room.

Volunteering to support other women is perhaps the best way you can turn your negative experience into a positive one though, particularly if you have been supported yourself though charity volunteers. Get in touch with PSS or the HER Foundation to volunteer your support, and they will be able to advise you how else you can get involved and help them.

Becoming a parent is the best thing I've ever done. It's given me a passion for life and love which I never imagined could exist. My enjoyment and passion for hard work has changed beyond recognition, as has my understanding of it. My appreciation for the important things in life is far more acute now, such as my health, and that of my family. My appreciation for sleep, as with any parent is deep! But I appreciate detail like waking up in the night and not feeling sick. I appreciate my ability to brush my teeth without retching or vomiting every night now. I appreciate being able to kiss and cuddle my children without finding the smell of them stomach turning. I appreciate every day I have with them, although some of those days it's not until long after they are in bed and I have a glass of wine in my hand that I appreciate it. But most of all, I appreciate my voice - when I was sick I couldn't defend myself at all, it was like I was mute, I couldn't speak out without being sick. I felt so weak, helpless, and pathetic. Now I can shout at the top of my voice, not just for myself but for the women suffering now. And that's what I've done and I'm doing and I'm going to carry on doing... and one day, Alfie and Patrick and Órlaith will be old enough to understand the work I do and they will be proud.

Caitlin, HG Survivor and author

Part IV

Resources and Appendix

APPENDIX 1

Resources, Websites, and Where To Get Help

The website that accompanies this book is *www.SpewingMummy.co.uk.* It is authored by Caitlin Dean and provides further information, support, and blog posts to help you through your pregnancy. There are also items you can download such as an HG Hero Certificate and a hyperemesis pregnancy calendar to help you through the long 9 months. You can also find links to products you can buy online such as Ketostix, rehydration salts, sick bags, etc.

Hyperemesis Gravidarum Organisations and Websites

Pregnancy Sickness Support (PSS) is the main UK Charity to help women and their carers with all degrees of Pregnancy Sickness. *Www.PregnancySicknessSupport.org.uk* tel: **024 7638 2020**

PSS provides a peer support network, loads of information leaflets, research and references, information for HCPs, and lots more. They also have a forum for online support and to connect with other sufferers.

Hyperemesis Education and Research Foundation (HER) is the main charity in North America and has a worldwide network of volunteers to provide support to sufferers. They can also help you locate an 'HG friendly' doctor near you. *Www.helpher.org*

Beyond Morning Sickness is a book written by Ashli Foshee McCall, the original HG book. It has provided support and information to countless thousands of women across the world and was very much the inspiration for this book. Her webmasters, Lyle Brooks and Natalie Mitchell, now match women with volunteers as soon as they make contact and can help source good doctors in America. They work closely with the HER Foundation and personally fund the provision of HG books to women who can't afford to buy them. *www.beyondmorningsickness.com/*

In the Netherlands, there is a website providing information and support *www.steunpunthg.nl/wordpress/*

In Canada, the **Motherisk** programme supports women with NVP and HG.

www.motherisk.org/women/index.jsp

Pregnancy Sickness SOS is a UK website run by Margaret O'Hara. She provides vast amounts of research and information in an accessible format https://sites.google.com/site/pregnancysicknesssos/

IV at Home Service

Sirona Care and Health is the NHS contracted community care company which nurse Emma Moxham works for and is pioneering the IV at Home service for women with HG. You can read about the service and contact them via their website: *www.sirona-cic.org.uk/news/2014/06/two-sirona-nurses-shortlisted-for-national-award/*

Termination/Abortion Support, Information, and Services

Marie Stopes International provides safe, supportive and non-judgmental advice and help from an expert clinic. They have a 24-hour helpline 0845 300 8090. Their website in the United Kingdom is *www.mariestopes.org.uk*.

The British Pregnancy Advisory Service (BPAS) also provides information, support, and abortion services. Their helpline is 03457 304030 in the United Kingdom or +44 1789 508211 from outside the United Kingdom. Their website is *www.bpas.org*

Mental Health Help

Mind is a national charity supporting all mental illness. They can provide help in a crisis and give further advice about help local to you. They support perinatal and postnatal mental health issues also. *www.mind.org.uk*

The British Association for Counselling and Psychotherapy is an organisation which can help you find a therapist or counsellor in your area. *www.bacp.co.uk/*

The Black Dog Tribe is a social networking platform for people with mental health condition. They offer support and help and a safe community. *Www.blackdogtribe.com*

In the South West of England, the **Angela Harrison Trust** provides support, information, and education about peri and postnatal depression. *www.help-4mums.org*

The Perinatal Illness UK Charity offers support and help for all mental or emotional ill health during and after pregnancy well worth getting in touch with if you need help. *www.pni-uk.com/*

Employment Help and Information

Gov.uk has a good explanation of the employee's rights.

www.gov.uk/time-off-for-dependants/your-rights

Info on eligibility and entitlement to parental leave can be found here:

www.gov.uk/parental-leave

The Citizens Advice Bureau has a number of fact sheets on employment rights including ones on pregnancy and maternity discrimination and unfair dismissal. These are available on their website *www.adviceguide.org.uk*. You may also wish to contact CAB for advice if you are experiencing problems at work as a result of your NVP/HG. Citizens Advice, ACAS *www.acas.org.uk*

Maternity Action is a charity which provides advice and information sheets on maternity rights and benefits *www.maternityaction.org.uk*. They also have a helpline 0845 600 8533.

Relationship and marriage guidance counselling

Relate is the leading UK relationship counselling service and provides sex therapy for couples also. You obviously don't need to be married to access their services and if you have financial difficulties they can provided help with costs of counselling sessions. The website is *www.relate.org.uk/*

Adoption and Fostering Help and Information

The British Association for Adoption and Fostering (BAAF) is one of the best places to start when you are looking for information about adoption and fostering. *www.baaf.org.uk*

The Adoption Social is an online community of adoption bloggers and home of The Weekly Adoption Shout Out where bloggers link up their own posts about life as adoptive parents. It is a great way of reading the ups and downs of family life and what it means to adopt a child. – *theadoptionsocial.com*

If you choose to either adopt or foster, you have two choices: you can apply directly through your local authority or you can apply through an independent agency who work with the local authority but can offer you different support options throughout your journey. The choice is completely up to you, and it's best to research all your options and contact a few agencies before making up your mind who to register with. BAAF have a list of independent agencies, which includes well-known names such as **Barnardos** (*www.barnardos.org.uk*) and **Action for Children** (*www.actionforchildren.org.uk*) as well as smaller agencies who work within a certain region only.

Amanda and her husband have personally contacted the **Independent Foster Care Agency, Foster Care Associates** (*www.thefca.co.uk/*) and have had a very positive experience so far. The staff are happy to call you for a chat about what fostering entails and answer any questions you may have. And as a large independent agency with 20 years experience and local teams in 50 towns throughout the UK, they are a good place to start.

Support for One Child Families

There are extensive links to support blogs and articles on the subject of one child families on Amanda Shortman's blog *www.thefamilypatch.com*

Childcare Links

If you employ a nanny to look after your children you will need to pay thier tax and provide them with payslips, an employment contract and so on. Nanny Tax is a company which you can instruct to do all of that on your behalf. There are a number of similar agencies to shop around but Caitlin has had personal experience with **Nanny Tax** while suffering HG and would recommend their service. Their website is *www.nannytax.co.uk*

Generally it is a good idea to ask locally for recommendations for childcare services, agencies, nurseries and so on. However, if you are short of time or don't know where to ask locally then **Childcare.co.uk** is a leading UK website helping parents locate local services. *www.childcare.co.uk*

Activity Ideas for Toddlers

Adventures of Adam is a toddler activity idea blog run by PSS trustee and

HG survivor Emma Edwards. She has a dedicated section for activities easy for mums suffering HG to entertain children at home whilst ill. Planned to have the most distraction for the child with the minimum amount of effort from mum. *Www.adventuresofadam.co.uk/hyperemesis-gravidarum/*

APPENDIX 2

Useful Charts and Tables

PUQE Scoring

In the table below, mark the answer to each question which best describes your own experience, and then use the scores next to each of your answers to give you a final 'score'. By doing this regularly, you can assess the effectiveness of the treatments and your progress.

Pregnancy Unique Quantification of Emesis and Vomiting Score (PUQE) – over 24 Hours	
In the last 24 hours, for how long have you felt nauseated of sick to your stomach?	Please circle the one answer
Not at all	1
1 hour or less	2
2–3 hours	3
4–6 hours	4
More than 6 hours	5
In the last 24 hours, have you vomited or thrown up?	Please circle the one answer
I did not throw up	1
1 to 2	2
3 to 4	3
5 to 6	4
7 or more times	5
In the last 24 hours, how many times have you had retching or dry heaves without bringing anything up?	Please circle the one answer
No times	1
1 to 2	2
3 to 4	3
5 to 6	4
7 or more times	5
On a scale of 1–6, how would you rate your nausea and/or vomiting today, if 1 is acceptable and 6 is extremely debilitating?	Please circle the one answer 1 2 3 4 5

Weekly Fluid Balance Chart:

To use this chart, use a regular cup/bottle/mug that you know how much it holds and can estimate how much you have had. If you use a mug that holds 200 ml and you drink one and a half during the morning, you'll have an intake of 300 ml (include ice lollies and jellies too). To monitor output, use a measuring jug to monitor your urine output. If you need to monitor vomit output, you can either use a vessel which you can estimate quantity in or use kitchen scales (1 mg = 1 ml) but don't forget to delete the weight of the bowl.

At the end of 24 hours, add up the totals and minus the output from the input to work out the balance.

	Morning 6 a.m.–12 p.m.		Afternoon 12 p.m.–6 p.m.		Night 6 p.m.–6 a.m.		Totals for 24 hours		
	Intake	Output	Intake	Output	Intake	Output	Intake	Output	Balance +/-
Day 1									
Day 2									
Day 3									
Day 4									
Day 5									
Day 6									
Day 7									

Weekly Drug Chart:

If you find it hard to keep on top of what to take when, particularly if you are drowsy, then ask your partner to fill this chart in and set alarms on your phone for medication time. Tick when you've taken your dose.

	Morning		Lunchtime		Tea time		Bedtime	
	Medication and dose	Taken ✓	Medication and dose	Taken ✓	Medication and dose	Taken ✓	Medication and dose	Taken ✓
Day 1								
Day 2								
Day 3								
Day 4								
Day 5								
Day 6								
Day 7								

GLOSSARY

Abortion – The deliberate ending of a pregnancy either by a medical or surgical procedure, resulting in the death of the foetus either before, during, or just after the procedure.

Anti-emetics – Medications which reduce the symptoms of nausea and vomiting. Different anti-emetic medications work in different ways to reduce symptoms.

Central Catheter or Central Line – A catheter (tube) line that is inserted into a large vein (usually the superior vena cava) in the neck area or near the heart. It is done for long-term access to give fluids, medication, or total parental nutrition. Blood samples can also be taken from the site.

Dehydration – Loss of essential fluid and salts required for normal body functioning. It occurs when you lose more fluid than you take on.

Electrolytes – Essential salts and minerals needed to conduct electrical impulses in the body. Electrolytes such as sodium chloride, potassium, calcium, and sodium bicarbonate are needed for humans. They control the fluid balance of the body and are required for almost every major biochemical reaction in the body such as muscle contraction and energy generation.

Emesis – Vomiting

Enteral Nutrition – It is a system of feeding (or giving medications) making use of the natural digestion process of the GIT. Enteral nutrition is generally preferable to parenteral nutrition, which is only used when the GI tract must be avoided.

Fluid Balance – Maintaining the correct amount of fluid in the body. It is the continuance of the fluid input and output of the body. Fluid balance can alter with disease and illness and a poor fluid balance can be indicative of dehydration and poor management of hyperemesis.

Gestation – The time the foetus is developing in the uterus from conception until birth; generally it is measured in weeks and days from LMP (see LMP)

GIT – Gastrointestinal Tract. The organ system responsible for consuming (ie. eating) and digesting food, absorbing nutrients, and expelling waste. It is divided into the upper and lower gastrointestinal tracts commonly defined as the stomach and intestine respectively.

GP – General practitioner, your doctor at your local surgery. Often the first port of call for women in the United Kingdom.

Hyperemesis Gravidarum – hyper – excessive, emesis – vomiting, gravidarum – of pregnancy. Hyperemesis gravidarum is an extreme form of pregnancy sickness and a dangerous complication of pregnancy. Characterised by extreme nausea and vomiting, rapid weight loss, and dehydration, hyperemesis requires treatment and careful medical management.

Intramuscular Injection – An injection given into the muscle, larger volumes of liquid can be given compared to subcutaneous injection

Intravenous Therapy (IV) – Also known as a drip, IV therapy is a short tube going into a vein generally in the hand, wrist, or elbow. It is used to give fluid replacement and medications.

Ketones – Chemicals which build up when the body needs to break down fats and fatty acids to use as fuel. This is most likely to occur when the body does not get enough sugar or carbohydrates. In HG management, urine is tested for the presence of ketones as an indication of dehydration and malnutrition.

LMP – Last menstrual period. The first day of your last period before conception. Generally used as the date to measure gestation from, although conception will actually have occurred approximately 2 weeks after this date.

Malnutrition – The condition that develops when the body does not get the right amount of the vitamins, minerals, and other nutrients it needs to maintain adequate organ function.

Naso Gastric Feeding Tube (NG) – This involves the insertion of a plastic tube (nasogastric tube or NG tube) through the nose, past the throat, and down into the stomach. For medications or small amounts of liquid, a syringe is used and injected into the tube. For feeding through an NG tube, a gravity is employed, with a liquid feed solution placed higher than the patient's stomach. Sometimes the tube is connected to an electronic pump which can control and measure the patient's intake and signal any interruption in the feeding.

Nausea – Feeling sick

Parenteral Nutrition – It is the provision of nutrition (or giving medication) into the body through a route which is not through the gastrointestinal tract (i.e. mouth or rectum). Usually given through a vein, intravenous infusion. Other parenteral routes of medication administration include injection, implantation, or through the skin

Percutaneous Endoscopic Gastrostomy (PEG) – This is a medical procedure in which a tube (PEG tube) is passed into a patient's stomach through the abdominal wall using endoscopy. This provides enteral nutrition despite bypassing the mouth. The PEG procedure does not require a general anaesthetic; mild sedation is typically used. PEG tubes may also be extended into the small intestines by passing a jejunal extension tube (PEG-J tube) through the PEG tube and into the jejunum via the pylorus.

Peripherally Inserted Central Catheter (PICC) – A long catheter (tube) which is inserted in a peripheral vein often at the elbow and is fed along the vein so that the end sits in the superior vena cava just by the heart. Like a central line, this is done for long-term access to administer fluids, medication, or total parental nutrition.

Post Traumatic Stress Disorder (PTSD) – A psychological reaction that can occur after a highly stressful, sometimes prolonged event. It is usually characterized by depression, anxiety, flashbacks, recurrent nightmares, and avoidance of reminders of the event. Due to the prolonged and intense nature of hyperemesis gravidarum, there are increasing reports of PTSD in sufferers.

Ptyalism – Excessive saliva production, a common symptom of hyperemesis gravidarum.

Subcutaneous Injection – A small injection given under the skin

Suppository – A medication which is given in the rectum or vagina. Useful in hyperemesis when oral medication is not tolerated

Teratogenic – Substances or agents that can interfere with normal embryonic development and cause birth defects

Termination – See Abortion

Total Parental Nutrition (TPN) – A complete nutrition delivered IV or via a peripherally inserted central catheter (PICC) or central catheter. Given to women who are completely unable to tolerate oral nutrition or in addition to oral nutrition in prolonged severe hyperemesis gravidarum.

spewing mummy

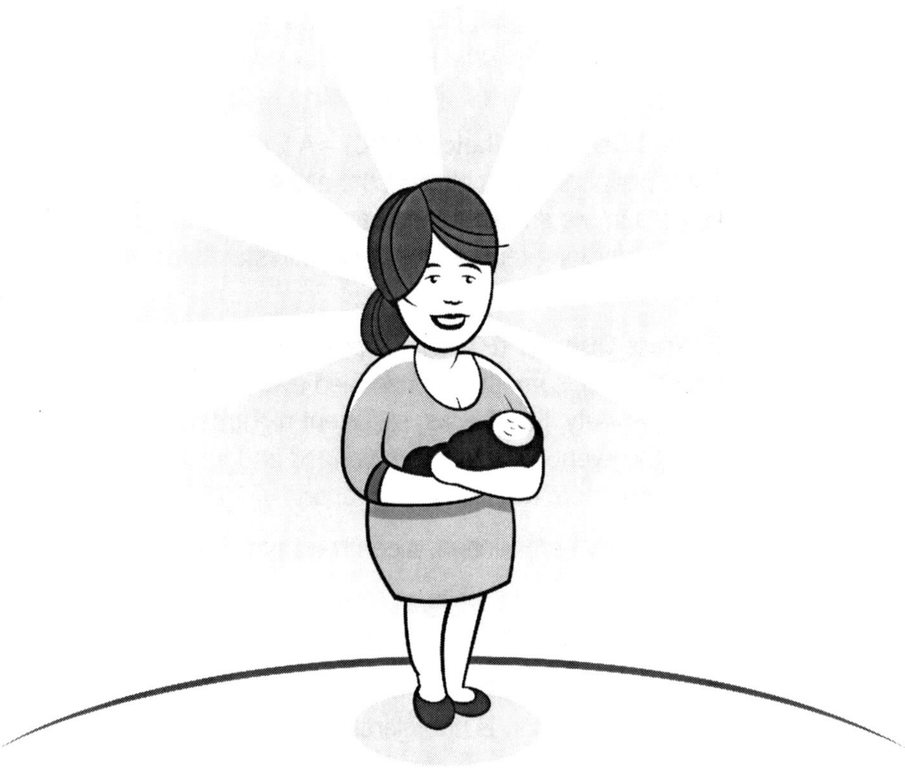

Index

Lightning Source UK Ltd.
Milton Keynes UK
UKOW04f1917051014

239678UK00013B/223/P